I0882125

HARRY'S COSMETICOLOGY
9TH EDITION

FOCUS BOOKS

ART AND SCIENCE OF FORMULATING COSMETIC PRODUCTS

ISBN: 978-08206-0199-1

Harry's Cosmeticology

9th Edition

© 2015 Chemical Publishing Co., Inc. All rights reserved.

No part of this publication may be reproduced, stored in a retrieval system or transmitted in any form or by any means, electronic, mechanical, photocopying, recording, scanning or otherwise, except as permitted under Sections 107 or 108 of the 1976 United States Copyright Act, without either the prior written permission of the Publisher. Requests to the Publisher for permission should be addressed to the Publisher, Chemical Publishing Company, through email at info@chemical-publishing.com.

The publisher, editors and authors make no representations or warranties with respect to the accuracy or completeness of the contents of this work and specifically disclaim all warranties, including without limitation,warranties of fitness for a particular purpose.

Volume One - ISBN: 978-0-8206-01762
Volume Two - ISBN: 978-0-8206-01779
Volume Three - ISBN: 978-0-8206-01786
eBook - ISBN: 978-0-8206-01793

First Edition

Chemical Publishing Company

www.chemical-publishing.com

Printed in the United States of America

A Note from the Publisher:

The new 9th edition of Harry's Cosmeticology is available as a 3 volume set containing over 2600 pages of new information on the recent changes in the cosmetic and personal care products industry.

Chemical Publishing is now offering key parts of the title for those interested in a particular subject area covered in the book.

Harry's Cosmeticology 9th Edition has developed a new line of titles called "Focus Books" for this purpose.

"Focus Books" are a series of selected chapters that can be used as a reference guide for partial subject areas covered in the parent text.

Because the chapters have been taken from the original individual volumes, the reader will find that the pages have not been renumbered in standard order starting from page one, moving forward, but rather they have been left in the original format so that the information will flow chronologically, although the pages may in fact not be numbered as so.

The benefit of leaving the page numbers as they were taken from the original text is that the reader will be able to use the Table of Contents and page numbers referenced within the Focus Book to find the desired content and we have tried to keep the chapter segments in the same order in which you would find them in the master text.

The full 3 volume Trilogy of Harry's Cosmeticology 9th Edition can be purchased through Chemical Publishing Company at www.chemical-publishing.com or through any major online retailer. It is also available in Ebook format through Kindle or as mobi, or ePub available directly from the publisher.

www.chemical-publishing.com

Our webpage featuring Authors, Reviews and other information about the 9th edition:

www.harryscosmeticology.com

About the Editor-in-Chief

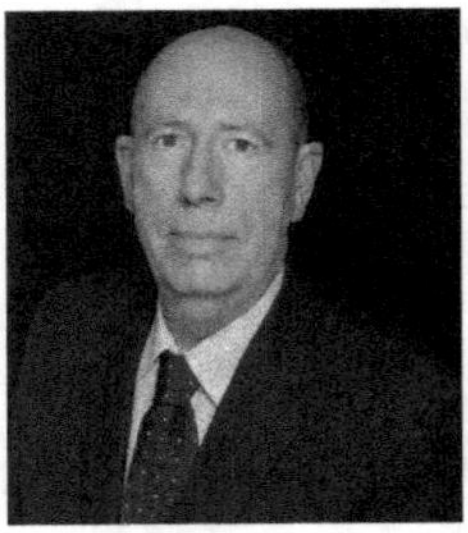

Meyer R. Rosen

CChem, CPC, CChE, CFEI, DABFE, DABFET, FAIC

Meyer R. Rosen is President of Interactive Consulting, Inc. (www.chemicalconsult.com). He is a Thought-Leader and expert in the field of Technical Marketing and multi-industry Technology Transfer Applications including, but not limited to: cosmetics and personal care, applied rheology, applied surface and interfacial chemistry, polymers, organosilicones, professional editing and custom preparation of Mind-Maps® for the organization and presentation of complex information.

Mr. Rosen is a Chartered Chemist and Fellow of the Royal Society of Chemistry (London); a Fellow of the American Institute of Chemists and both a Nationally Certified Professional Chemist and Certified Professional Chemical Engineer. He is a member of the U.S. Society of Cosmetic Chemists (SCC) & the American Institute of Chemical Engineers. Meyer serves as an Advisor for David Smith, Executive Director of the SCC Advisory Committee. He is also Editor for U.S. & Canada and Editor-in-Chief for North and Latin America for Euro Cosmetics Magazine in Germany. Mr. Rosen is Editor of the Delivery System Handbook for Personal Care and Cosmetic Products and Editor-in-Chief of Harry's Cosmeticology, 9th Ed.

Meyer served for six years as the Chief Scientific Advisor and Director of Technical Programming for United Business Media's (UBM) HBA Technical Conferences. He a former Director of the American Institute of Chemists, past Vice President of the Association of Consulting Chemists and has served on the Scientific Advisory Board of Supply Side West/East: Virgo Publications. Mr. Rosen is also the Founder, Organizer and co-moderator for HBA's Annual International Safety, Regulatory and Certification Symposia.

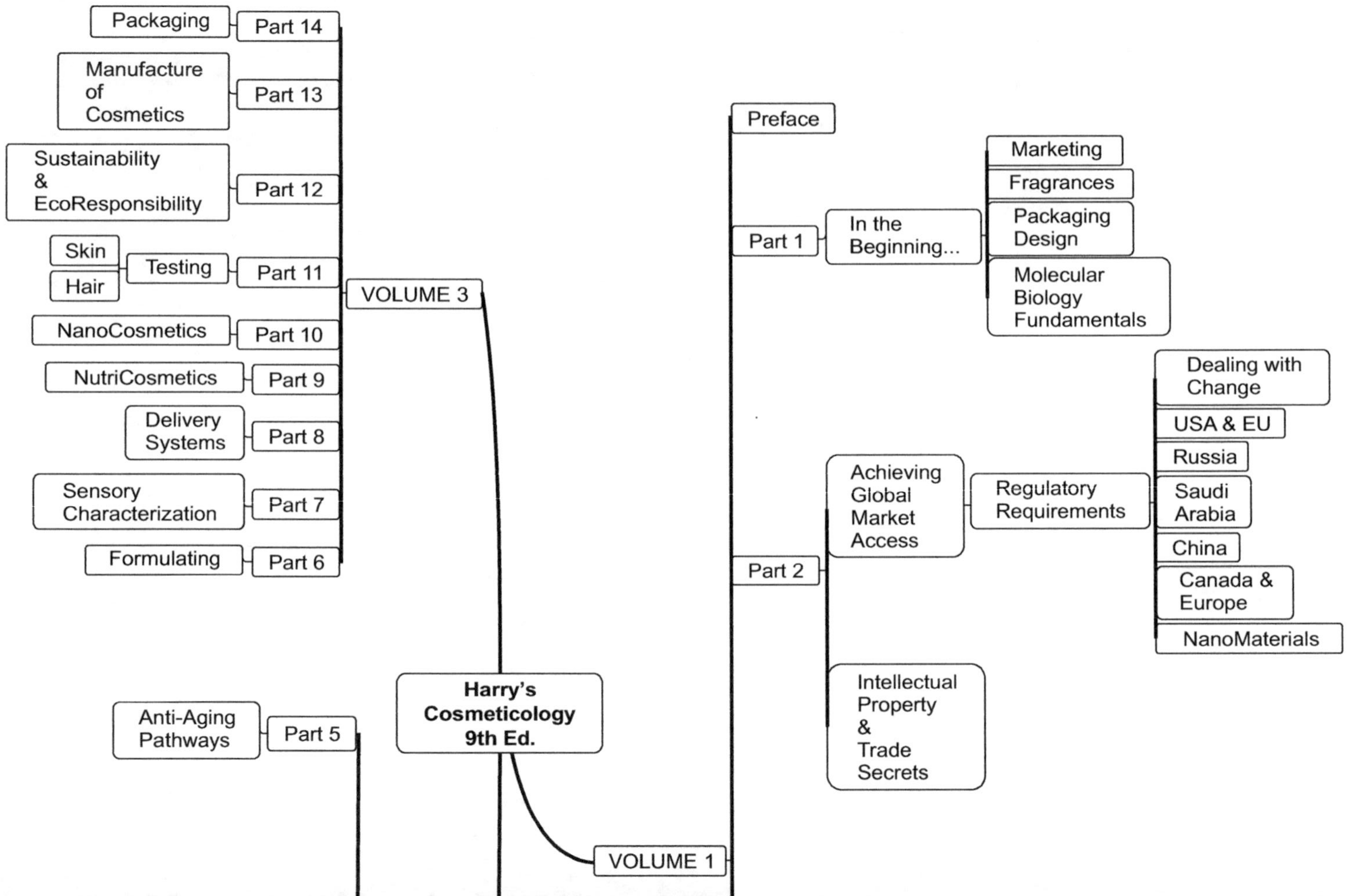
Harry's Cosmeticology 9th Ed.
VOLUME 1
Preface
Part 1
In the Beginning...
Marketing
Fragrances
Packaging Design
Molecular Biology Fundamentals
Part 2
Achieving Global Market Access
Regulatory Requirements
Dealing with Change
USA & EU
Russia
Saudi Arabia
China
Canada & Europe
NanoMaterials
Intellectual Property & Trade Secrets
Part 5
Anti-Aging Pathways
VOLUME 3
Part 6
Formulating
Part 7
Sensory Characterization
Part 8
Delivery Systems
Part 9
NutriCosmetics
Part 10
NanoCosmetics
Part 11
Testing
Skin
Hair
Part 12
Sustainability & EcoResponsibility
Part 13
Manufacture of Cosmetics
Part 14
Packaging

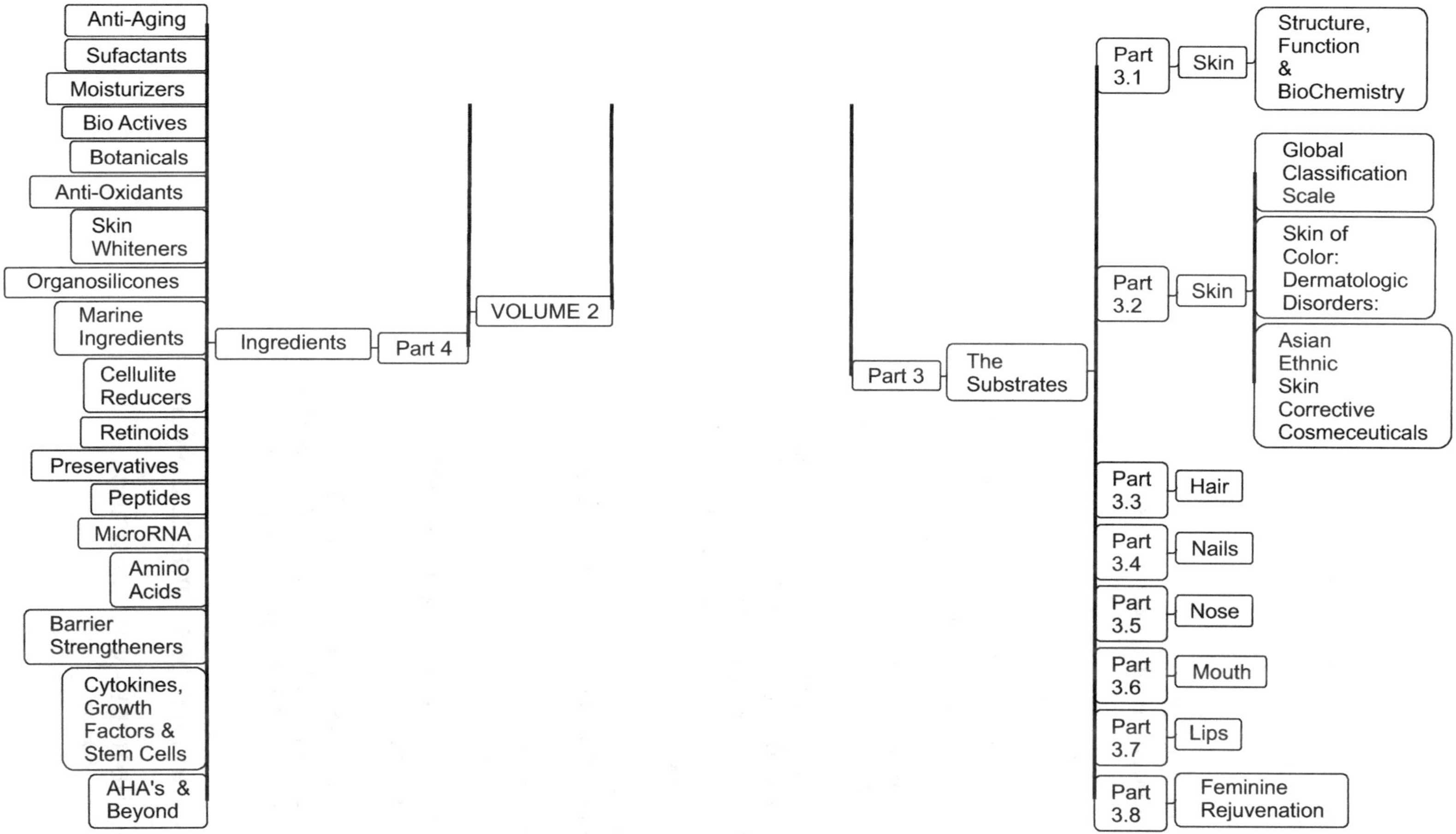

VOLUME 2
Part 4
Ingredients
Anti-Aging
Sufactants
Moisturizers
Bio Actives
Botanicals
Anti-Oxidants
Skin Whiteners
Organosilicones
Marine Ingredients
Cellulite Reducers
Retinoids
Preservatives
Peptides
MicroRNA
Amino Acids
Barrier Strengtheners
Cytokines, Growth Factors & Stem Cells
AHA's & Beyond
Part 3
The Substrates
Part 3.1
Skin
Structure, Function & BioChemistry
Part 3.2
Skin
Global Classification Scale
Skin of Color: Dermatologic Disorders:
Asian Ethnic Skin Corrective Cosmeceuticals
Part 3.3
Hair
Part 3.4
Nails
Part 3.5
Nose
Part 3.6
Mouth
Part 3.7
Lips
Part 3.8
Feminine Rejuvenation

AUTHORS:

FORMULATING COSMETICS AND PERSONAL CARE PRODUCTS

Editor:

Charles Warren
President, Charles F. Warren Consulting Inc

Contributors:
Eva Patel, Skin Rx
Gurpreet (Gogi) Sangha, CEO of G.S. Cosmeceutical
Mark Lees, Ph.D., M.S., CIDESCO Diplomate
Germain Puccetti, Ashland Chemical
Nevine Issa, and Hani Fares Ph. D
Carrie Shipley, Grain Processing Corporation
Padmaja Prem, VP of Combe's Global Research

SKIN LIGHTENING, WHITENING, AND BRIGHTENING: AN OVERVIEW OF APPROACHES, KEY INGREDIENTS, AND FORMULATIONS FOR ENHANCING SKIN APPEARANCE AND CORRECTING/MINIMIZING COMMON SKIN PIGMENTATION DISORDERS

Authors:
Eva Patel & Gurpreet (Gogi) Sangha

SUNSCREENS
Charles Warren

ANTIPERSPIRANTS / DEODORANTS
Charles Warren

ACNE, OILY, AND AGING SKIN PRODUCT FORMULATION ESTHETIC MANAGEMENT OF ACNE-PRONE AND CLOG-PRONE SKIN

Author
Mark Lees, Ph.D., M.S., CIDESCO Diplomate

FACE AND BODY - MASKS / SCRUBS
Charles Warren

AUTHORS

SHAVING PREPARATIONS: PRE AND POST
Charles Warren

PIGMENTED COSMETICS

COLOR COSMETICS: AN INTRODUCTION TO FORMULATION AND APPROACHES FOR MASCARAS, FOUNDATIONS AND LIPSTICKS

Authors
Germain Puccetti, Nevine Issa, and Hani Fares

HAIR CARE

SHAMPOOS INGREDIENTS, FORMULATION AND EFFICACY EVALUATION

Author
Carrie Shipley, Applications Scientist, Grain Processing Corporation

HAIR STYLING
Charles Warren

SPECIALTY STYLING PRODUCTS
Charles Warren

PERMANENT WAVING
Charles Warren

CONDITIONERS/TREATMENTS
Charles Warren

REACTIVE HAIR CARE PRODUCTS
Charles Warren

FORMULA/PRODUCT DEVELOPMENT FROM THE FORMULATOR'S VIEWPOINT (EXPECTATIONS, INITIAL PROTOTYPES, FINAL PROTOTYPES)
Charles Warren

AUTHORS

ORAL CARE: FORMULATING PRODUCTS
AND PRACTICES FOR HEALTH AND BEAUTY

Editor:
Caren M. Barnes
Professor Coordinator of Clinical Research
University of Nebraska Medical Center College of Dentistry

Contributors:

Chi Shing Wong
Member, Product Development Group
Colgate-Palmolive Global Toothbrush Division

James G Masters, Ph.D.
Director in the Research and Development Division
Colgate-Palmolive Company

Shira Pilch, Ph.D.
Associate Director: Research and Development Division
Colgate-Palmolive Company

Michael Prencipe, Ph.D.
Director in the Research and Development Division
Colgate-Palmolive Company

PART 6 FORMULATING COSMETICS AND PERSONAL CARE PRODUCTS

Editor:

Charles Warren
President, Charles F. Warren Consulting Inc

Contributors:

Charles Warren Charles F. Warren Consulting Inc.
Eva Patel, Skin Rx

Gurpreet (Gogi) Sangha, CEO of G.S. Cosmeceutical

Mark Lees, Ph.D., M.S., CIDESCO Diplomate
Germain Puccetti, Ashland Chemical

Nevine Issa, and Hani Fares Ph.D.
Carrie Shipley, Grain Processing Corporation

Padmaja Prem, VP of Combe's Global Research

SKIN CARE
OVERVIEW

PART 6.1

FORMULATING WISDOM CATEGORY BY CATEGORY

Author: Charles Warren

PART 6.2

SKIN LIGHTENING, WHITENING, AND BRIGHTENING: AN OVERVIEW OF APPROACHES, KEY INGREDIENTS, AND FORMULATIONS FOR ENHANCING SKIN APPEARANCE AND CORRECTING/MINIMIZING COMMON SKIN PIGMENTATION DISORDERS

Authors: Eva Patel and Gogi Sangha

TABLE OF CONTENTS

PART 6.3

SUNSCREENS 1312

Author Charles Warren

PART 6.4

ANTIPERSPIRANTS / DEODORANTS 1314

Author Charles Warren

PART 6.5

ACNE, OILY, AD AGING SKIN PRODUCT FORMULATION

Author Mark Lees

TABLE OF CONTENTS

PART 6.6

FACE AND BODY - MASKS / SCRUBS

Author Charles Warren

TABLE OF CONTENTS

PART 6.7

SHAVING PREPARATIONS: PRE AND POST

Author Charles Warren

TABLE OF CONTENTS

PIGMENTED COSMETICS

PART 6.8

COLOR COSMETICS: AN INTRODUCTION TO FORMULATION AND APPROACHES FOR MASCARAS, FOUNDATIONS AND LIPSTICKS

Authors: Germain Puccetti, Nevine Issa, and Hani Fares

TABLE OF CONTENTS

SHAMPOOS INGREDIENTS, FORMULATION AND EFFICACY EVALUATION

Author Carrie Shipley, Applications Scientist, Grain Processing Corporation

TABLE OF CONTENTS

PART 6.11

HAIR STYLING

Author Charles Warren

PART 6.12

SPECIALTY STYLING PRODUCTS 1402

Author Charles Warren

PART 6.13

PERMANENT WAVING 1403

Author Charles Warren

PART 6.14

CONDITIONERS/TREATMENTS 1404

Author Charles Warren

PART 6.15

HAIR COLORANTS AND PROTECTION

Author: Padmaja Prem Vice President, Research & Development
Combe Incorporated, 1101 Westchester Avenue
White Plains, NY 10604

TABLE OF CONTENTS

PART 6.16

REACTIVE HAIR CARE PRODUCTS

Author Charles Warren

TABLE OF CONTENTS

PART 6.17

FORMULA/PRODUCT DEVELOPMENT FROM THE FORMULATOR'S VIEWPOINT (EXPECTATIONS, INITIAL PROTOTYPES, FINAL PROTOTYPES)

Author Charles Warren

TABLE OF CONTENTS

ORAL CARE: FORMULATING PRODUCTS AND PRACTICES FOR HEALTH AND BEAUTY

Editor:
Caren M. Barnes
Professor Coordinator of Clinical Research
University of Nebraska Medical Center College of Dentistry

Contributors:
Chi Shing Wong
Member, Product Development Group
Colgate-Palmolive Global Toothbrush Division

James G Masters, Ph.D.
Director in the Research and Development Division
Colgate-Palmolive Company

Shira Pilch, Ph.D.
Associate Director: Research and Development Division
Colgate-Palmolive Company

Michael Prencipe, Ph.D.
Director in the Research and Development Division
Colgate-Palmolive Company

TABLE OF CONTENTS:

PART 6

ART AND SCIENCE OF FORMULATING COSMETIC PRODUCTS

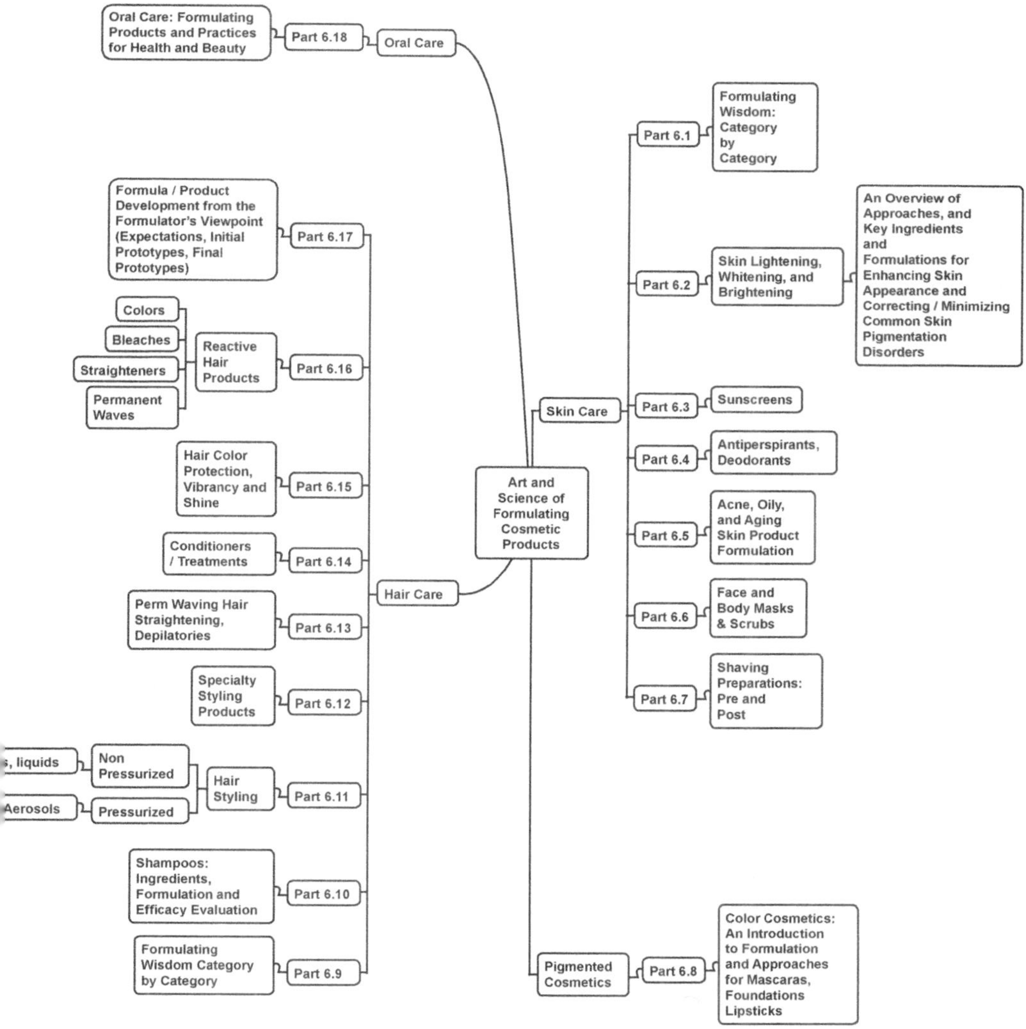

PART 6

FORMULATING COSMETICS AND PERSONAL CARE PRODUCTS

Editor
Charles Warren
President, Charles F. Warren Consulting Inc

Contributors:
Charles Warren,
Eva Patel, Skin Rx
Gurpreet (Gogi) Sangha, CEO of G.S. Cosmeceutical
Mark Lees, Ph.D., M.S., CIDESCO Diplomate
Germain Puccetti, Ashland Chemical
Nevine Issa, and Hani Fares Ph. D
Carrie Shipley, Grain Processing Corporation
Padmaja Prem, VP of Combe's Global Research

ABSTRACT

An overview of the science and art of formulating personal care products follows. Included are: specific product category overviews of hair and skin care products, detailed formulating information on selected product categories (e.g., shampoo) and an overview of the formula/product development process from the formulator's viewpoint.

TABLE OF CONTENTS

SKIN CARE

OVERVIEW

Exactly what is a "formulator"?

First and foremost, a formulator is a good scientist. A formulator has to have a good technical sense and a fundamental understanding of chemistry, biology, physics, statistics, and consumer sciences. The deeper and more complete the technical understanding, the better and more creative the formulating can be.

A formulator needs to understand the chemical relationships among the raw materials being used in whatever category the formulating is being done. Understanding the chemical function of the raw materials and their interactions with other raw materials allows the formulator to choose the best combination(s) for the particular end formula.

Likewise, a formulator has to understand the physics and physical properties of the desired end product – dictated by the category, the manufacturing requirements, the filling and dispensing properties and, most importantly, the physical characteristics desired by the ultimate consumer.

The formulator needs to understand the medium upon which the formulation is to be used—hair or skin and how that medium is impacted (positively and negatively) by the application of the particular formula. In addition, the formulator must understand the potential microbiological perils that can be introduced into the formula and the safest, most effective ways of preventing those contaminations from affecting the formula.

The formulator needs to understand how the formula is put together during manufacture and filling and how those operations impact the properties of the formulation. Additionally, the formulator needs to understand the relationship between the formula and the primary packaging, with special attention to how the formula will be dispensed from the package. Many formulators have had the unpleasant surprise of watching their formula become too thick as it is forced through a small orifice or, worst of all, cannot be dispensed from the package selected.

Consumer science is important for the formulator because the consumer is the ultimate judge of a product and, ultimately, its success in the marketplace. Understanding consumer testing and the statistical analysis of consumer data will always be of great benefit to the formulator. Dealing with consumer expectations is always challenging, but those expectations are extremely important to formulation and the ultimate marketing of a successful product.

Secondly, a good formulator needs to be an artist. Translating the "wish-list" from Marketing or the Consumer into a tangible consumer product is truly an art. Understanding the aesthetic requirements and the particular combinations of raw materials that deliver against those requirements is definitely an artistic endeavor and one that a good formulator must really take the time to pursue.

So, a formulator is a combination of scientist and artist, a good observer of both technical and aesthetic properties, a good listener to all interested partners—Marketing, the Consumer, Manufacturing, etc., and an objective and unbiased evaluator of information.

A formulator needs to understand the category in which the formula is being developed

In skin care, the categories are usually split between hand/body and facial products. In hand/body care there are cleansers, moisturizers, and a group of miscellaneous products, such as sunscreens. In facial care there are cleansers/scrubs, moisturizers, and treatments, such as acne treatments, fine-line and wrinkle treatments, masques, etc. There are other groups of products also, such as perfumes/fragrances, pigmented cosmetics, nail products, and products related to shaving and depilatory products.

In hair care, the categories are: shampoo, conditioner/treatments, styling and reactive products. The formulator also needs to understand the targeted consumer within the category. A general market shampoo for European hair would have different technical and aesthetic requirements than a shampoo for African/Caribbean hair or a shampoo for Asian hair.

An understanding of the existing environment, individual company, and competitive arena for each category is a good starting point. If the formulator is working for a company, a thorough understanding of the existing formulations within the category is important in understanding the palette of raw materials and familiarity with manufacturing. A review of the competitors in the category will provide insight into what is having success in the category and where there may be formulating opportunities.

This section will be devoted to providing assistance to the new formulator and review and refreshment for the experienced formulator.

PART 6.1

FORMULATING WISDOM – CATEGORY BY CATEGORY

Author

Charles Warren

The skin is the largest organ of the human body. Below the outermost layer (stratum corneum) the skin is a living, biologically active organ. Unlike hair, healthy skin can repair itself and every 28 days actually replaces itself. It is the barrier between the internal body (75–80% water) and the external environment (significantly lower water content) and all of the perils it faces from that same external environment.

When formulating for skin care, there are two major categories: Hand and Body Care and Facial Care.

Hand/Body

Cleansers

The general categories of body and hand cleansers are soaps, bodywashes, and liquid hand washes. The function of all of these is to cleanse the body and hands of excess oils, particulates, and other substances adhering to or residing on the skin. Soaps are a special category, while bodywashes and liquid hand cleansers are very similar in form and composition.

The classic definition of a soap is an ionic salt of a long-chain fatty acid. A long-chain fatty acid, such as stearic acid, is neutralized with an alkali material to a stearate. When neutralized with sodium hydroxide, sodium stearate results; with ammonium hydroxide, ammonium stearate, etc. These stearates will emulsify the oils on the skin and adhere to particulates and then allow them to be rinsed away with water. Formulating and manufacturing soaps is a specialized endeavor and is usually handled by suppliers or manufacturers highly skilled in this medium.

Bodywashes and liquid hand cleansers are more prevalent and more reasonably formulated and manufactured by personal care formulators/manufacturers. In general, these are aqueous solutions of primary surfactants (e.g., laureth sulfate), secondary surfactants (e.g., betaines), foam modifiers (e.g., cocamide MEA), conditioning agents (e.g., hydroxypropyl trimonium chloride), aesthetic modifiers such as sodium chloride (viscosity), color and fragrance, and microbiological preservatives. If the product is to be opaque or pearlescent, materials such as glycol stearate can also be used. Once an acceptable base formulation of surfactants and modifiers is identified, a wide variety of variables can be developed by changing colors, fragrances, and other additives to support positions and claims. These products can be easily formulated to dispense from tubes, bottles, through pumps, etc.

Moisturizers

The largest groups in this category are the hand and body lotions. These formulations are typically oil-in-water emulsions. Their primary function is to develop a light, oily layer on the surface of the skin to prevent water from leaving the lower layers of the skin, causing the surface to dry, flake, and develop a dull appearance. In addition, the other ingredients will help bind and retain moisture in the surface layers of the skin, leave the skin feeling soft and pliable, and impart a pleasing look and feel to the skin for an extended period of time.

A general overview of the ingredients used in these products would include:

- Water – the mobile phase of the emulsion
- Glycerin – a humectant that will reside in the stratum corneum and bind and hold water to itself
- Isopropyl palmitate – a light oily material to lubricate the skin and help occlude for water retention
- Petrolatum – the best occlusive agent to prevent trans-epidermal water loss (TEWL) and provide body and stiffness to the lotion
- Silicones/cyclosilicones – help improve spreadability and feel of the lotion on the skin
- Distearyldimonium chloride – a skin conditioner to help make the skin feel soft and pliable
- Cetyl alcohol/cetearyl alcohol/ceteth-20 – common emulsifiers to hold the oil droplets in the emulsion

In addition, various other fatty esters, cationic polymers, and thickening agents can be used to improve the texture and feel of the lotion.

A word of caution – Certain claims related to protection and "healing" can quickly move a formula from a cosmetic product into the realm of over-the-counter drugs (OTC). OTC drugs have very specific requirements related to the levels of the active ingredient (e.g., dimethicone), the claims and exact wording of the allowable claims, stability and packaging testing, labeling, and manufacturing. A prudent formulator will review formulas and claims with Regulatory and/or Legal groups to ensure compliance.

SKIN LIGHTENING, WHITENING, AND BRIGHTENING: AN OVERVIEW OF APPROACHES, KEY INGREDIENTS, AND FORMULATIONS FOR ENHANCING SKIN APPEARANCE AND CORRECTING/MINIMIZING COMMON SKIN PIGMENTATION DISORDERS

Authors

Eva Patel & Gurpreet (Gogi) Sangha

ABSTRACT:

Skin-lightening products form a major segment in the cosmeceuticals market worldwide; and they carry with them the promise of flawless-appearing skin. This demand for "skin-fairness" products stems from the desire to eliminate hyper-pigmentation, melasma, and post-inflammatory hyperpigmentation as well as a consumer interest to lighten overall skin tone through the use of skin lighteners, whiteners, and brighteners.

The continually growing demand for skin tone corrective treatments by the global beauty market has prompted scientists to develop an array of natural and synthetic raw materials that work on various pathways of skin pigmentation. Most skin lighteners currently in use are of botanical or natural origin and have multi-functional topical benefits. Such materials can also act as free radical scavengers for skin that has been over exposed to UVA and UVB solar radiation. These specialty ingredients can be formulated into topical solutions such as creams, serums, and lotions.

In the U.S., topical compositions containing hydroquinone are the only ones that regulations allow to make a skin-whitening and -lightening claim. Such compositions have been classified by the U.S. FDA as a drug. Many botanical, natural, and synthetic ingredients are available that may produce results similar to those of hydroquinone; however, current regulations covering compositions containing such ingredients are only allowed to make the claim of "skin brightening."

TABLE OF CONTENTS

Skin Lightening, Whitening, Brightening

Skin lightening has become a significant trend attracting the interest of technologists, product developers, and marketing/business leaders. Today, women, and even men, want to alter the tone and appearance of their skin to meet current regional standards of beauty or to address an underlying medical or cosmetic condition. Amazingly, skin whitening has become increasingly popular.

In the USA many people desire flawless and even-toned complexions; however, this is not the case in Asia. In this geographical area, *it is a cultural issue* that one has fair skin as it is a sign of beauty, wealth, and status. An article in *The Economist* titled "The Line of Beauty" (August 27th, 2011) suggests that good-looking people are more likely to succeed, be accepted by their peers, and get higher-paying jobs. In many countries, socioeconomic status depends on your skin color, as for example in India and Mexico. In India even your marriage is based on skin color, and the rising skin-tone consciousness continues to grow rapidly. From an epidemiological point of view, we find this trend-to-whiteness fascinating in view of the well-recognized global shift in the population towards darker-skin peoples.

6.2.1 DEFINITIONS

Skin Lightening & Whitening/Skin Bleaching: A common drug claim for OTC/RX products containing Hydroquinone, as this is the only skin-lightening active ingredient that is recognized by the U.S. FDA.

Skin Brightening: Brightening is a term used throughout the skin care industry to classify formulations that brighten uneven skin tone and contain alternatives to hydroquinone. These alternatives can include botanicals, natural ingredients, peptides, and vitamins. Natural skin lighteners are also considered multifunctional ingredients that provide multiple benefits for the skin.

Hyperpigmentation/Melasma: Overproduction of melanin in the skin that is denoted by dark spots or patches

Hypopigmentation/Vitiligo: Areas of the skin that have lost their pigment completely when there are no longer functioning melanocytes in that area to create pigment, leaving white spots or patches on the skin

Melanogenesis: The process of melanin being formed in the melanocyte located at the dermal/epidermal junction in the skin

Melanin: The substance that gives our skin its color/pigment. This natural pigment is our skin's protective shield against UV aggression. Dark skin tones contain more melanin in their skin and lighter skin tones have less melanin.

6.2.2 COMMON SKIN PIGMENTATION DISORDERS

1. Melasma/Chloasma – A condition that is typically induced from hormones internally. Also known as a pregnancy mask because most cases are seen in women postpartum. This condition can also be induced from menopause and even certain medications. MSH (melanocyte-stimulating hormone) is a natural hormone in our bodies and is linked to pigmentation and hyperpigmentation development in individuals with Melasma/Chloasma.
2. Post-Inflammatory Hyperpigmentation – This condition can be seen in the skin after inflammation has been present. Most commonly found in acneic skin conditions, this term is a broad category and includes "acne prone, reactive, oily skin type," that experiences persistent breakouts and also post–aggressive skin care treatments or medical procedures.
3. Sun Damage – Sun is the number one trigger for hyperpigmentation, causing sun spots from years of excessive exposure to the ultraviolet rays. These are also known as photo damage or age spots.

6.2.3 TRIGGERS FOR HYPERPIGMENTATION

1. Sun (UVA/UVB rays, environmental damages, free radicals)
2. Hormones (internal unbalance, pregnancy, menopause)
3. Inflammation (blemishes, acne, injury, laser treatment, heat, medical procedures, chemical procedures)
4. Oral Medications (diuretics, birth control pills, antibiotics, anti-depressants, etc.)
5. Alcohol (aftershave, colognes, perfumes)

6.2.4 PATHWAY TO HYPERPIGMENTATION:

Formation of melanin is influenced by many different factors including genetics, certain medications, diet, and environmental factors. In today's market there are many different types of skin-brightening ingredients that target the process of pigment formation via multiple modes of action. The term "tyrosinase inhibitor" has been used widely in the market to define a skin-brightening active. This term is true for certain active ingredients; however, not all skin-brightening ingredients directly interfere with the catalyzing of the tyrosinase enzyme. Tyrosinase is a copper-containing enzyme where copper and oxygen act as catalysts. Kojic acid is a specific ingredient that directly affects tyrosinase by chelating the copper within the enzyme-active site. The antagonist effect of kojic acid results in an inactive form of the tyrosinase enzyme that no longer allows for the production of melanin. As seen in Figure 6.2, the tyrosinase enzyme is a key component for melanin to be produced and should always be targeted in an effective skin-lightening formulation. Another area of focus is to look at other biochemical processes involved in melanogenesis. By looking at the "Pathway to Hyperpigmentation" we can analyze the different stages in which active ingredients can be targeted to more effectively control pigment production and produce the most visible changes in skin tone and appearance.

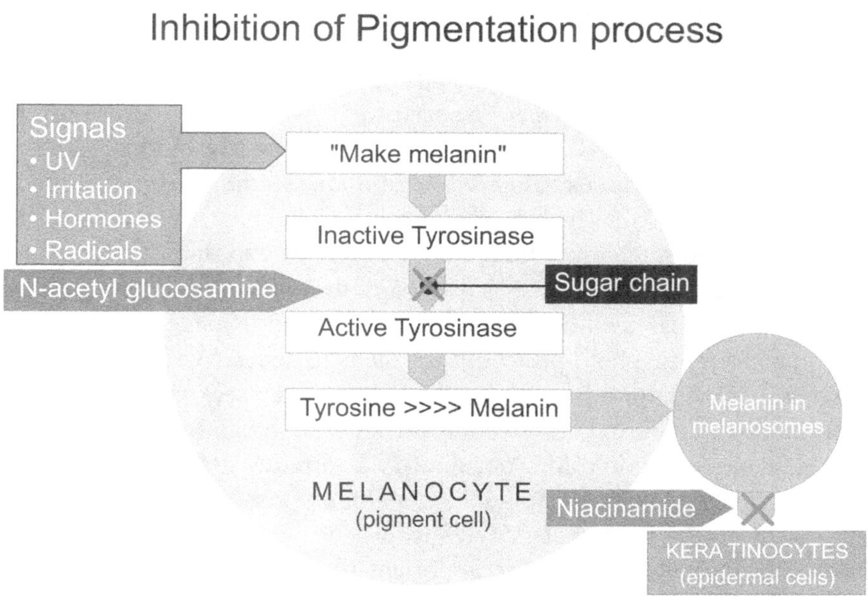

Figure 6.2. Inhibition of Pigmentation Process

1. One of the first things to occur in the skin along the pathway to hyperpigmentation is the generation of tyrosine, which is an amino acid naturally occurring in our bodies. Tyrosine is then converted to L-dopa by an enzyme called tyrosinase.
2. Tyrosinase catalyzes with L-dopa and converts it into dopaquinone.
3. Melanin is then created and put into our melanosomes.
4. Melanosomes are transferred into the keratinocytes, also known as our skin cells, which then continue on their journey up through the epidermis where they eventually are bio-converted to corneocytes and appear on the surface of the skin.

Besides the aforementioned pathways there are other ways to help suppress melanin formation. **Melanogenesis** is a complex process of oxidative stages in which topical antioxidants are useful to combat hyperpigmentation. Many antioxidants have skin-brightening properties that also provide multifunctional benefits. Antioxidants help to reduce hyperpigmentation by scavenging free radicals that can be a precursor to hyperpigmentation. Another example is MSH, melanin-stimulating hormone (melanotropin), which can be inhibited by certain ingredients. (1)

A variety of other avenues are used to increase cell turnover, which will provide skin-brightening results, as well as remove pigment from the surface for an instantly brighter glow. Alpha Hydroxy Acids (AHA) and kertolytic enzymes, such as papaya and bromalein, help to exfoliate surface stratum corneum cells to promote brighter, more even-tone complexion. Finally, the importance of using a UV absorber is crucial in order to see results and maintain those results from skin-lightening actives. Hyperpigmentation due to UV exposure can be addressed by using preventative measures, which include applying a physical/chemical broad-spectrum sunscreen regularly when exposed to UV radiation. The use of broad-spectrum photo-stable UVA/UVB sunscreens and protective clothing are one of the best ways to enjoy sun exposure while minimizing the deleterious effects of UV aggression on the skin. There are a number of companies who have woven UV absorbent fibers into protective clothing to prevent sun exposure. These items can be wide-brimmed hats, long-sleeved shirts, pants that when coupled with the use of UV-protectant sunglasses all help to protect the skin for extended times outdoors. The best commonsense photo-protective advice is to take cover in the shade when the sun's rays are strongest between 10 a.m. and 4 p.m. Seek cover indoors or at least in a shaded spot during those hours when the UV index is at its most intense. Even though sun protection does not directly interfere with the pigment formation process, it helps to block UV radiation and limit post-sun exposure erythema, which are key triggers for melanocytes to produce melanin. The technological advances described above are quite important for formulators of sun-protection products since they describe the skin hyperpigment formation process and how we can target different pathways to inhibit it.

6.2.5 FORMULATING INGREDIENTS—A PLETHORA OF RAW MATERIALS AND HOW THEY COME INTO PLAY

Actiwhite® PW LS 9860: A synergistic skin-lightening complex based on pea extract and a sugar ester. This innovative mechanism has dual mode of action for optimal skin-lightening effect. The material does not affect the color of the formulation, has excellent compatibility and stability, and can be formulated in a broad pH range, even in combination with AHAs. This active component contains a high capacity to decrease melanogenesis. It works to decrease tyrosinase activity and reduce melanosomes from maturing.

Supplier: BASF Personal Care Ingredients

Arbutin: A potent antioxidant that is an extract from the bearberry plant. Arbutin works by inhibiting the activity of the tyrosinase enzyme to reduce hyper-pigmentation and protects the skin against free radical damage. Arbutin suppresses the activity of tyrosinase enzyme and prevents melanosome from forming. Arbutin is chemically similar to hydroquinone.

Bearberry (Uva ursi) Extract: This plant leaf extract contains arbutin and methyl arbutin, both hydroquinone derivatives with skin-whitening properties.

β-White™ (Oligopeptide-68): An encapsulated peptide that mimics the signaling protein of the tyrosinase enzyme to reduce the amount of signaling proteins that activate tyrosinase to produce melanin. According to Unipex Innovations, an *in vitro* comparative study showed that β-White induced significant skin-lightening effects on 23 Asian volunteers with at least one hyperpigmented spot after four weeks.

Supplier: Lucas Meyer Cosmetics

Chromabright™ (Dimethylmethoxy Chromanyl Palmitate): An advanced engineered amino acid that fights against photo-aging. Chromabright reduces dopaquinone so that it cannot convert into DOPA, therefore inhibiting another pathway to melanin formation.

Supplier: Lipotec

Ethyl Ascorbic Acid: A novel vitamin C derivative with excellent whitening, anti-oxidation, radicals-scavenging and collagen-increasing effect. Its stability is superior to other ascorbic acid derivatives. It is widely used in skin care products, especially desirable for whitening and anti-ageing products.

Supplier: EME Ltd.

Glycolic Acid: Known as one of the most-used alpha hydroxy acids in the industry. Glycolic acid is naturally derived from sugar cane. It helps to speed up cell turnover and removes pigmentation from the outer layers of the skin to instantly brighten skin.

Hexylresorcinol: A widely known ingredient that has been used in the food industry for preservation and in oral and topical applications. Hexylresorcinol has antibacterial properties, and inhibits the tyrosinase enzyme to give a brighter, more even skin tone. **(Symwhite: Symrise)**

Hydroquinone: Hydroquinone is a very well-known ingredient to bleach the skin. Working through a variety of mechanisms, this ingredient reduces the formation of melanosomes and even induces melanocyte cytotoxicity. Hydroquinone is the only ingredient approved by the U.S. FDA for skin-whitening claims.

Kojic Acid: Derived from mushrooms and other species of fungus. This form of kojic acid is water soluble and inhibits tyrosinase enzyme by blocking copper from catalyzing with tyrosinase, which results in an inactive enzyme. This effective brightening agent also provides antibacterial properties.

Kojic Acid Dipalmitate: Derived from mushrooms and other species of fungus. This form of kojic acid is oil soluble and inhibits tyrosinase by chelating the copper contained within the tyrosinase enzyme resulting in a deactivated enzyme. This effective brightening agent also provides antibacterial properties. Compared to kojic acid, it offers improved efficacy and stability, and is easier to make with water-based formulations.

Esterases in the skin hydrolyze the ester bond, cleaving the fatty chain off kojic DP and allowing bioavailable KA to be liberated. (2)

Lactic Acid: A well-known alpha hydroxy acid that contains skin-brightening properties. Mostly derived from sour milk and sugars, this active exfoliates to instantly brighten skin and suppresses tyrosinase.

Licorice Root: This well-known extract inhibits the tyrosinase enzyme without causing cytotoxicity. This material also reduces UV-induced hyperpigmentation and inflammation in the skin, which are precursors to hyperpigmentation.

Lumiskin: Made up of triglycerides, this active ingredient acts as a competitive antagonist to the tyrosinase enzyme and suppresses the tyrosinase activity. Lumiskin inhibits calcium flow into the cells and thus reduces tyrosinase activity (stabilizes it in its inactive form) and melanogenesis.

Supplier: Croda

Lumisphere™: This complex combines Diacetyl Boldine and manganese titanium dioxide (TiO2-Mn) to instantly and gradually brighten the skin. Lumisphere, the Diacetyl Boldine (DAB) stabilizes tyrosinase in its inactive form. It also contains TiO2Mn, which can absorb UVA and UVB and neutralizes free radicals, resulting in a more even skin tone.

Supplier: Croda

Magnesium Ascorbyl Phosphate: Is a stable water-soluble derivative of vitamin C. It is an excellent antioxidant, stimulates collagen production, and is well known for its melanin-inhibiting properties.

Supplier: Caribbean Natural Products Inc.

The bioconversion needed to liberate the active form L-ascorbic acid phosphatase enzymes within the skin change this pro-form into bioavailable ascorbic acid.

References:

Mia Campos et al.: Ascorbic Acid and Its Derivatives in Cosmetic Formulations, Cosmetics and Toiletries, 11,59-62 (2000)

Melanostatine®-5: A skin-brightening peptide that is created in a lab to also inhibit the alpha-melanocyte-stimulating hormone (MSH). This active ingredient does not allow the hormone to signal the melanocyte to produce melanin, thus preventing and suppressing hyperpigmentation.

Supplier: Lucas Meyer (aka Unipex)

Meiritage: Combination of plant extracts used in Traditional Chinese Medicine: Atractylodes macrocephalae, Bupleurum falcatum, and Astragalus membranaceus roots, to prevent wrinkles and even out the complexion.

Supplier: Croda/Sederma

Mulberry (Morus bombycis): The root and bark extracts of the mulberry plant might also play a role in inhibiting the tyrosinase enzyme that converts tyrosine into melanin's precursors. Mulberry contains arbutin, which inhibits melanin production.

O.D.A. White: Octadecenedioic acid is obtained by a biofermentation process from natural and vegetable oleic acid. O.D.A. White helps to inhibit the entire pathway of melanin synthesis from the nucleus of the melanocyte by reducing levels of tyrosinase mRNA. This active ingredient treats all types of pigmentation, even ethnic skin. The use of antioxidants in combination with ODA White is recommended.

Supplier: Croda

Phytic Acid: Most commonly found in grains, bran, and seeds. Phytic acid has been used as an antioxidant for years in the food industry. It works via a chelation mode of action by blocking the copper contained within the tyrosinase enzyme from catalyzing to form melanin.

Regu®-Fade: A nature identical trans-resveratrol ingredient based on a biofermentation that increases cell longevity and reduces inflammation. Resveratrol is made up of a polyphenol and has strong antioxidant properties to protect skin against free radicals and environmental damages. REGU®-FADE helps reduce the appearance of skin pigmentation as demonstrated in clinical and *in vitro* studies, resulting in noticeably brighter, younger-looking skin.

Supplier: DSM Nutritional Products, Inc.

Sepiwhite MSH (Undecylenoyl Phenylalanine): A highly advanced engineered active ingredient that inhibits the alpha-melanocyte-stimulating hormone (MSH).

Supplier: Seppic

Tetrahexyldecyl Ascorbate: Most commonly derived from citrus components. Advancements of vitamin C have been engineered to contain multiple benefits with greater efficacy and stability than L-Ascorbic Acid alone. Tetrahexyldecyl Ascorbate works as an antioxidant in the skin that also encourages brighter skin tone. This engineered form allows for better penetration into the skin and even suppresses melanogenesis up to 80% by inhibiting tyrosinase enzyme.

Tyrostat™ (rurnex occidentalis extract): Derived from plants native to Canada. Extracts of this plant have strong effect to inhibit the tyrosinase enzyme, resulting in a more even skin tone. Unipex screens the plant material for tyrosinase activity before it enters the extraction process to guarantee optimal activity. *In vitro* and clinical data have demonstrated that Tyrostat™ safely reduces skin pigmentation and erythema for a more uniform complexion. It also has outstanding results in the reduction of the appearance of age spots.

Supplier: Lucas Meyer Cosmetics

WONDERLIGHT™: An active ingredient of plant origin (hop cone), a regulator of the pigment disorders by inhibiting the cytokine GM-CSF (activator of melanogenesis).

Supplier: Croda/Sederma

Vitamin A: Also known as Retinol, is a multifunctional active ingredient that promotes youthful and even-toned skin. Vitamin A inhibits tyrosinase activity and reduces the amounts of melanosomes that are produced. This ingredient will also help to increase cell turnover and increase penetration of skin-brightening actives into the skin. When using a product containing Vitamin A and or its derivatives, it is mandatory to use in the evening only and accompany it with a broad-spectrum UVA/UVB SPF 30 during the day.

It is clear from the extensive array of the skin-whitening ingredients described above that formulators have great flexibility in selecting optimal agents and combinations of those agents to formulate products that address the global interest in skin whitening and brightening.

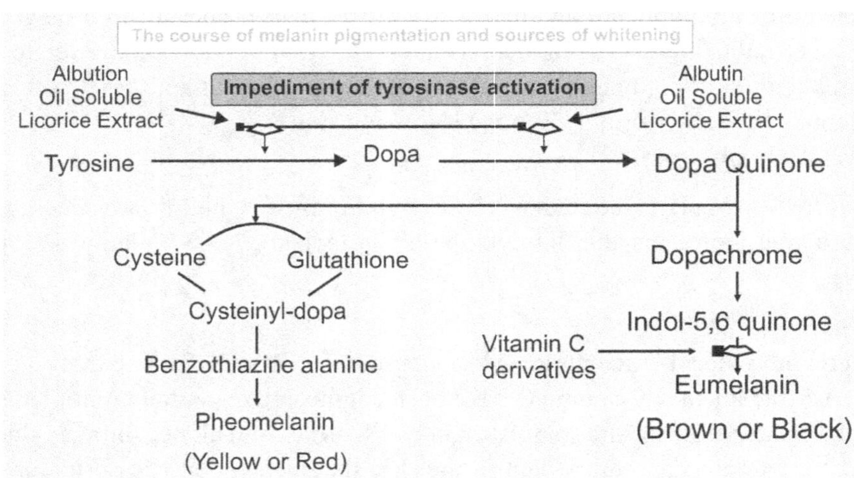

Figure 6.2.1

6.2.6 FORMULATIONS FOR INDIVIDUAL SKIN CONDITIONS

Whitening Cream

Ingredient Listing: Aqua (Water), Glycerin, Isopropyl Palmitate, Cetyl Alcohol, Stearyl Alcohol, Cetearyl Alcohol, Alpha Arbutin, Butylene Glycol, Kojic Dipalmitate, Dicetyl Phosphate, Ceteth-10 Phosphate, Hydrogenated Lecithin, Sodium Oleate, Oligopeptide-68, Glycyrrhiza Glabra (Licorice) Root Extract, Dimethylmethoxy Chromanyl Palmitate (Chromabright Proposed INCI), Sodium Metabisulfite, Sodium Sulfite, Phenoxyethanol, Sodium Ascorbyl Phosphate, Hexylresorcinol, Potassium Sorbate, Sodium Benzoate, Xanthan gum, Disodium EDTA

PHASE INGREDIENT/SUPPLIER

Phase A	**wt/%**
Cetearyl Alcohol (and) Ceteareth 18 Symrise (2/014200 Dragowax S.E.)	8.00
Cetearyl Octanoate (and) Isopropyl Myristate Symrise (2/066210 PCL Liquid)	3.00
Mineral Oil Exxon Mobil (Marcol 82)	5.00
Octyl Octanoate Symrise (2/044115 Dragoxat EH)	1.00
Dimethicone Dow corning (200/350 cs)	1.00
Phase B	
Deionized Water	75.45
Xanthan Gum (Keltrol F)	0.10
Pentylene Glycol Symrise (2/016020 Hydrolite-5)	3.00
Glycerin BP	1.20
Phenoxyethanol (and) Methylparaben (and) Ethylparaben (and) Isobutylparaben (and) Propylparaben (and) Butylparaben Symrise (2/060140 Dragocide Liquid)	0.80
Sodium Hydroxide 1% Solution	0.10
C Tyrostat™-11 Unipex innovations	1.00
D Fragrance O/H 64583 The Vert Symrise	0.30

PROCEDURE:

1. Disperse the Keltrol F in water.
2. Heat Phase A and B separately to 80°C.
3. Add Phase B into A under vigorous stirring and homogenize.
4. Allow batch to cool to 45°C and add Tyrostat-11 and homogenize.
5. Add the fragrance at 35°C.

Skin-Brightening & Anti-Aging Moisturizing Lotion with Resveratrol

Phase A	**wt/%**
Water (aqua) (deionized)	70.98
Versene 220 Crystals (Dow Chemical) (Tetrasodium EDTA)	0.02
Rhodicare XC (Rhodia) (Xanthan gum)	0.20
Propylene Glycol USP (Lyondell)	3.00
CoSept PEP (HallStar) (Phenoxyethanol, methylparaben, ethylparaben, butylparaben, propylparaben, isobutylparaben)	0.60
Phase B	
HallStar GC (HallStar) (Caprylic/capric triglycerides)	5.00
BioChemica Jojoba Oil — Ultra Refined (HallStar) (Simmondsia chinensis [jojoba] seed oil)	3.00
BioChemica Sunflower Seed Oil (HallStar) (Helianthus annuus [sunflower] seed oil)	2.00
BioChemica Shea Butter — Ultra Refined (HallStar) (Butyrospermum parkii [shea butter])	3.00
HallStar GMS Pure (HallStar) (Glyceryl stearate)	0.32
HallStar GMS SE/AS (HallStar) (Glyceryl stearate, PEG-100 stearate)	3.00
HallStar TA-1618 Cetearyl Alcohol (HallStar) (Cetearyl alcohol)	0.70
SolaStay S1 (HallStar) (Ethylhexyl methoxycrylene)	4.00
RTD HC-40 (HallStar) (PEG-40 Hydrogenated castor oil)	1.00
Phase C	
BioChemica Vitamin E Natural (HallStar) (Tocopherol)	1.00
BHT (Merisol Antioxidants) (BHT)	0.08
Regu-Fade (DSM Nutritional) (Resveratrol)	0.10
Phase D	
MSS-500W (Kobo Products) (Silica)	2.00

PROCEDURE:

To a suitable vessel equipped with mixing, heating, and cooling capabilities, add phase A and start mixing. To a second-phase vessel equipped with heating and cooling capabilities, charge phase B. Mix phases A/B while heating to 70°–75°C. When phases A/B are at 70°–75°C, slowly add phase B to phase A while maintaining temperature and adequate mixing. Homogenize for 10 minutes and then resume mixing and start cooling. At 122°F (50°C) or lower, add phase C and D; mix well while recirculating through a pump/mill combination. Cool to ambient temperature and then add water as needed to bring to full batch mass. When again uniform, stop mixing, perform final quality-assurance checks, and package product.

PROPERTIES:

(25°C): Appearance—Light yellow lotion; viscosity (RV, T-D, 5, 20 & 100 rpm, cP)—10800, 3500 & 1120; pH—6.0.

Reference: The HallStar Company

Skin-Lightening Cream Gel with Alpha-Arbutin and DISMUTIN®-PF

Phase A	**wt/%**
Ethylhexyl Isononanoate (Pelemol 89/Phoenix Chemicals)	5.00
Isohexadecane (Arlamol HD/Uniqema)	2.00
Diethylhexyl Carbonate (Tegosoft DEC/Evonik)	5.00
Dimethicone (DC200fluid/200cts/Dow Corning)	1.00
Phase B	
Ammonium Acryloyldimethyltaurate & VP Copolymer (Arisoflex AVC/Clariant)	1.20
Phase C	
Deionized Water	68.90
Glycerin (Rita Glycerin USP/Rita)	5.00
DISMUTIN-PF	0.20
DIOCIDE	0.70
Phase D	
Deionized Water	10.00
ALPHA-ARBUTIN	1.00
Phase E	
Citric Acid (10% solution)	q.s. to pH 5

PROCEDURE:

1. Mix phase A together. Add phase B to phase A, mix until homogeneous.
2. Mix together phase C.
3. Premix phase D ingredients and add to phase C.
4. Add phase C/D to phase A/B. Homogenize to obtain a homogenous cream gel.

Reference: Centerchem, Inc.

High Protection SPF 30 Sunscreen with Skin-Lightening Properties

Phase A	**wt/%**
Parsol HMS (DSM) (Homosalate; USAN)	10.00
Parsol 1789 (DSM) (Butyl methoxydibenzoylmethane) (Avobenzone; USAN)	3.00
Parsol 340 (DSM) (Octocrylene) (octocrilene; USAN)	2.70
Parsol EHS (DSM) (Ethylhexyl salicylate Octisalate; USAN)	5.00

Parsol SLX (DSM) (Polysilicone-15)	0.99
Amphisol K (DSM) (Potassium cetyl phosphate)	2.00
Eusolex 4360 (Merck) (Benzophenone-3) (Oxybenzone; USAN)	6.00
Lanette O (Cognis Deutschland) (Cetearyl alcohol)	2.50
dl-alpha-Tocopherol (DSM) (Tocopherol)	0.20
Euxyl PE 9010 (Schülke & Mayr) (Phenoxyethanol & ethylhexylglycerin)	1.00
Cetiol CC (Cognis) (Dicaprylyl carbonate)	3.00
Finsolv TN (Innospec) (C12-15 alkyl benzoate)	3.00
Lipocire Na 10 Pastilles (Gattefossé) (Hydrogenated coco-glycerides)	1.00
Antaron V-216 (International Specialty Products) (VP/hexadecene copolymer)	1.00
Phase B	
1,3-Butylenglykol (Brenntag AG) (Butylene glycol)	3.00
Keltrol CG SF (CP Kelco) (Xanthan gum)	0.20
Edeta BD (BASF) (Disodium EDTA)	0.10
Water dem. (Aqua)	51.31
Phase C	
Orgasol Caresse (Atofina) (Polyamide-5)	2.00
Phase D	
Alpha-Arbutin (DSM)	2.00

PROCEDURE:

Heat phase A to 85°C while stirring. Heat phase B to 80°C and add to phase A while stirring and homogenizing the emulsion. Cool down the emulsion to 40°C, add phase C, and homogenize again.

PROPERTIES:

pH—5.56 ;Viscosity—14600 cps (Brookfield, RV4,10 rpm); SPF *in vivo*—34.0 *In vitro* UVAPF (Colipa 2007)—1.7; PA—UVAPF/SPF (30 labeled); >0.33—0.39; PFA: Critical Wavelength—376.0.

Reference: DSM Nutritional Products

Skin-Brightening Cream with Chromabright MFF

Phase A	**wt/%**
Deionized water	65.95
Ultrez 10 (Lubrizol)	0.15

1,3-butylene glycol	6.00
Hispagel 200 NS (Cognis Iberia)	10.00
Phase B	
Promulgen D (Lubrizol) (Cetearyl alcohol and ceteareth-20)	1.50
Cutina GMS-V NA (Cognis) (Glyceryl stearate)	1.25
Myrj 59 (Uniqema) (PEG-100 Stearate)	1.00
Fitoderm (Lipotec)	4.00
Tegosoft CT (Evonik) (Caprylic/capric triglyceride)	3.00
Lameform TGI (Cognis) (Polyglyceryl-3 diisostearate)	0.50
Phase C	
Tealan 99% (RITA) (Triethanolamine)	0.15
Deionized water	1.00
Phase D	
Chromabright MFF (Lipotec)	5.00
Diocide (Centerchem)	0.50

PRODEDURE:

Heat phase B to 75°C. Slowly add carbomer to phase A water and mix until uniform. Begin heating to 75°C. Add remaining phase A ingredients and mix until uniform. When both phases are at 75°C, add phase B to phase A under moderate mixing. Mix for 10 minutes. Begin cool down. At 50°C, add phase C as a solution. Mix until uniform. At 35°C, add phase D ingredients. Mix until uniform.

Reference: Centerchem, Inc.,

Age Spot Treatment Cream

Phase A	**wt/%**
Estol 3650 (Uniqema) (Glyceryl myristate)	2.50
Lanette 16 (Cognis) (Cetyl Alcohol)	2.50
Parsol EHS (DSM) (Ethylhexyl salicylate) (octisalate; USAN)	5.00
Parsol 1789 (DSM) (Butyl Methoxydibenzoylmethane) (Avobenzone; USAN)	2.00
Parsol 340 (DSM) (Octocrylene ; USAN)	1.70
Sweet almond oil (Gustav Heess) (Prunus amygdalus dulcis [sweet almond] oil)	2.00
Finsolv TN (Innospec) (C12-15 alkyl benzoate)	8.00
Butylated hydroxytoluene (Merck) (BHT)	0.05
dl-alpha Tocopheryl acetate (DSM) (Tocopheryl acetate)	1.00
Phenonip (Clariant) (Phenoxyethanol &	

methylparaben & ethylparaben & butylparaben & propylparaben & isobutylparaben)	0.80
Brij 72 (Uniqema) (Steareth-2)	2.00
Brij 721 (Uniqmea) (Steareth-21)	2.00
Dow Corning 345 Fluid (Dow Corning) (Cyclopentasiloxane & cyclohexasiloxane)	4.00
Phase B	
Water demineralized	45.35
(Merck) (Butylene glycol)	2.00
Glycerin (Cognis)	3.00
Edeta BD (BASF) (Disodium EDTA)	0.10
Keltrol CG-T (CP Kelco) (Xanthan gum)	0.20
Carbopol Ultrez 21 (Noveon) (Acrylates/ C10-30 alkyl acrylate crosspolymer)	0.25
Phase C	
Water demineralized	10.00
Stay-C 50 (DSM) (Sodium ascorbyl phosphate)	2.00
Niacinamide PC (DSM) (Niacinamide)	3.00
(Merck) (Sodium metabisulfite)	0.05

PROCEDURE:

Heat phase A up to 85°C; and also heat phase B up to 85°C. When both have the same temperature, add phase B to phase A while homogenizing intensively. Cool down the product to 35°C while stirring. Now add phase C and homogenize intensively again. It is generally recommended to use vacuum while producing the emulsion.

PROPERTIES:

pH—7.19; Viscosity—52800 cps (Brookfield, RV 6, 10 rpm).

Reference: DSM Nutritional Products

Brightening Lemon Under-Eye Crème

Phase A	**wt/%**
Water	q.s.
ABS White Willow Bark Extract Powder	2.00
(Salix alba [willow] bark extract) (Active Concepts) Glycerin	2.00
Dermofeel PA-3 (Kinetik Technologies) (Sodium phytate)	0.20
Ultrez 10 (Protameen) (Carbomer)	0.50

Phase B

Procol CS-20-D (Protameen) (Cetearyl alcohol [and] ceteareth-20)	3.00
Olive oil (Arista) (Olea europaea [olive] fruit oil)	1.00
Stearic Acid (RITA Corp.) (Stearic acid)	2.00
Jojoba Oil Clear (Arista) (Simmondsia chinensis [jojoba] seed oil)	1.00
RITA SA (RITA Corp.) (Stearyl alcohol)	1.50
Dermofeel BGC (Kinetik Technologies) (Butylene glycol dicaprylate/dicaprate)	1.00
Phase C	
ACB Bamboo Bioferment (Active Concepts) (Lactobacillus/arundinaria gigantea ferment extract)	1.00
Phase D	
ACB Lemon Peel Extract (Active Concepts) (Lactobacillus/citrus medica limonum [lemon] peel ferment extract [and] butylene glycol)	2.00
AC DermaPeptide Micro C (Active Concepts) (Saccharomyces/capsicum annum fruit ferment filtrate)	0.50
ACB Yogurt Dermal Respiratory Factor (Active Concepts) (Lactobacillus bulgaricus ferment filtrate)	5.00
Stabilized Vitamin C (Active Concepts) (Ascorbic acid)	0.50
Phase E	
Glycerin	5.00
AC Leucidal (Active Concepts) (Leconostoc kimchii [radish] root ferment filtrate)	0.50
Phase F	
Lavender and Vanilla Sage 302669 (American Flavors and Fragrances) (Fragrance)	0.25

PROCEDURE:

Phase A: Charge water into main beaker and begin propeller mixing. A vortex should form. Begin heating to 75°C. Sift in ABS white willow bark powder extract. Charge glycerin and dermofeel PA-3. Sift in Ultrez 10.

Phase B: In a separate container, blend ingredients and heat to 80°C. Once temperatures have been reached, add to main. Maintain temperature of 78°C and continue mixing for 15 minutes.

Phase C: Remove heat. Add at 60°C.

Phase D: Add each at 45°C. Slowly sift in stabilized vitamin C. Pre-blend and add to main.

Reference: Active Concepts

Skin-Lightening Gel

Phase A	**wt%**
Water	77.30
Natrosol 250 HHR (Hercules F) (Hydroxyethylcellulose)	1.50
Abil B 88183 (Degussa/Goldschmidt) (PEG/PPG-20/6 dimethicone)	2.00
Phase B	
Glycerin	3.00
Preservative	q.s.
Phase C	
NaOH 10% (Sodium hydroxide)	q.s. to pH 8.5
Citric acid	q.s. to pH 4-5
Phase D	
EDG Plus (Moellhausen S.p.A.) (Ethoxydiglycol)	5.0
Phase E	
Water	10.00
Alpha-Arbutin (Pentapharm)	1.00
Uvinul DS 49 (BASF) (Benzophenone-9)	0.20

PROCEDURE:

Disperse Natrosol 250 HHR in water, then add Abil B 88183. Mix phase B, then add it to phase A. Adjust the pH to approx. 8.5 with NaOH 10% to obtain a clear gel. Then adjust the pH to approx. 4.0–5.0 with citric acid. Add phase D under stirring. Add phase E and mix to obtain a homogeneous gel.

Reference: Centerchem, Inc.

Skin-Lightening Cream for Age Spots

Phase A	**wt/%**
Cremophor A6 (Ceteareth 6, stearyl alchohol)	2.50
Cremophor A25 (Ceteareth 25)	2.50

Cutina GMS V (Glyceryl stearate)	4.00
Lanette O (Cetearyl alcohol)	3.00
Stearic acid	1.00
Paraffin oil (Mineral oil)	10.00
Cetiol SN (Cetearyl isononanoate)	5.00
Vaseline white (Petrolatum white)	3.00
Abil-350 (Dimethicone)	4.00
Phase B	
Deionized water	51.10
Pentavitin (Centerchem, Pentapharm) (Saccharide isomerate)	5.00
Phase C	
Glycerin	3.00
Phenonip	0.50
Phase D	
Melfade J (Centerchem, Pentapharm) (Water, arctostaphylos uva ursi leaf extract, glycerin, magnesium ascorbyl phosphate)	5.00
Sodium metabisulfite	0.10
Phase E	
Fragrance (Chiara 0/238927)	0.30

PROCEDURE:

Heat the ingredients of fatty phase A to 70°C. Heat the ingredients of water phase B to 75°C. While stirring add phase B to phase A, cool to 50°C, homogenize and cool to 30°C. Then add phase C and stir cold. Finally, incorporate phases D and E one after the other and adjust the pH to 4.5.

Reference: Centerchem, Inc.

Age Spot Defense	**wt/%**
Deionized water	86.5
Hydrolite-5 (pentylene glycol)	5.00
Tego Cosmo C 250 (Degussa Goldschmidt PC) (1-methylhydantoine-2-imide)	0.10
Aerosil R 812 S VV 60 (Degussa AG Aerosils & Silanes) (silica silylate)	5.00
Dimethicone 20 cps	2.00

Abil B 8843 (Degussa Goldschmidt PC) (PEG-14 dimethicone)	0.50
Liquipar Oil (isobutylparaben [and] isopropylparaben [and] butylparaben)	0.15
Covagel (sodium carboxymethyl starch)	0.75

PROCEDURE:

Place water and Hydrolite-5 in a mixer; add Sericite FSE and Tego Cosmo C 250 while stirring. Disperse by homogenizing briefly. Add Aerosil R 812 S VV 60 while homogenizing and homogenize for another 10 minutes. Check for complete dispersion. Add dimethicone 20cps, Abil B 8843 and Liquipar Oil while stirring and stir for another two to three minutes. Add Covagel while stirring and stir for another 15 minutes.

Reference: Degussa Corp. Business Line Aerosil

6.2.7 CLAIMS/REGULATIONS IN USA

Skin-Lightening Claims for USA:

Definition of a skin-bleaching active ingredient, according to the U.S. Food & Drug Association (FDA), is an agent designed to bleach or otherwise lighten limited areas of hyperpigmented skin through the suppression of melanin pigment formation within skin cells.

Hydroquinone is the only skin-bleaching active ingredient recognized by the FDA. The active ingredient and its concentration in the product are as follows for OTC: Hydroquinone 1.5 to 2.0 percent. Any increased concentration over 2 percent is considered a prescription that needs to be prescribed by a doctor.

Label Claims:

Hydroquinone may be combined with any generally recognized safe and effective sunscreen active ingredient, provided that the product is labeled accordingly.

The labeling of the product must contain the established name of the drug. It should identify the product as a skin-bleaching agent, skin lightener, or skin bleaching, e.g., lotion, cream, gel, etc. The labeling of the product contains a statement of the indications that is limited to the following phrases: "For the gradual fading or lightening of dark discolorations/spots/areas/freckles/age spots." The label should also contain the appropriate warnings identified by the FDA.

For skin-lightening products that *do not* contain Hydroquinone, which are considered natural alternatives to hydroquinone, refrain from making any of the above label claims. These products contain other skin-brightening actives like kojic acid, brightening peptides, and licorice root extract. A common term used to describe these alternatives is "skin brightening," or you can say it helps to promote a more even skin tone. Only skin-lightening products that contain Hydroquinone can make skin-lightening claims because Hydroquinone is the only active ingredient that is actually recognized by the FDA as a skin-bleaching agent.

REFERENCES

1. Schallreuter KU, Moore J, Tobin DJ, Gibbons NJ, Marshall HS, Jenner T, et al. alpha-MSH can control the essential cofactor 6-tetrahydrobiopterin in melanogenesis. Ann NY Acad Sci. 1999; 885: 329–41.)
2. Sarmad Al-Edresi et al., In-vitro and in-vivo evaluation of a photo-protective kojic dipalmitate loaded into nano-creams. **Asian Journal of Pharmaceutical Sciences 2010, 5 (6): 251–265.** Supplier: Caribbean Natural Products Inc.

PART 6.3

SUNSCREENS

Author

Charles Warren

Sunscreens (for body)

Sunshine contains both UV A and UV B rays, which are harmful to the living cells in the skin. UV B radiation is the cause of sunburn ranging from cellular damage to painful skin reddening and in some cases blistering and peeling. UV A radiation is related to the degradation of the cells and destruction of collagen and elastin cells leading to premature aging of the skin with all of the attendant negative effects—wrinkling, leathery skin appearance, etc. Sunscreens are chemicals that absorb the UV radiation and prevent the radiation from reaching the cells within the skin.

In the United States, sunscreens are regulated under an OTC monograph that dictates allowable sunscreens and levels, testing requirements, claims, labeling requirements, etc. Other countries throughout the world have their own regulations related to allowable sunscreens, levels, claims, label requirements, etc., and all of these requirements are not consistent. Sunscreens, levels, and claims allowed in one country may not be allowed in another. Similarly, countries may have different required testing for claims, stability, safety, etc. Formulators should consult the appropriate regulatory/legal groups prior to initiating formulation to determine what is and is not allowed in the market(s) of interest, what testing (functionality, analytical, stability, safety, etc.) may be required and any special registrations or preapprovals needed.

Sunscreens for the body are usually found in the following forms: cream/lotion, nonpressurized pump spray, or pressurized aerosol spray. The sunscreen ingredients for these products are chosen to: a) deliver the desired SPF rating; and b) be stable in the base formula for the desired form. The combination of and concentration of the individual sunscreens are what provide the desired SPF rating. Commonly employed sunscreens are: avobenzone, octisalate, oxybenzone, homosalate, octocrylene, titanium dioxide, and zinc oxide (the latter two actually blocking the UV radiation). The allowable levels of each sunscreen are indicated in the sunscreen monograph. Additional sunscreens are also included in the monograph. Suppliers of the various sunscreens can be very helpful in suggesting appropriate combinations and levels to achieve a particular SPF rating.

The creams and lotions are generally oil-in-water emulsions, composed of a water phase including water, glycerin, a thickening polymer (e.g., carbomer or the copolymers, such as acrylates/octylacrylamide copolymer), glycerin, C_{12-15} alcohol benzoate, and so on. The oil phase can include fatty alcohols (e.g., cetyl alcohol), fatty acids (e.g., stearic acid), dimethicone, distearyldimonium chloride, cyclopentasiloxane, and so on. The emulsification system, usually incorporated in the oil phase, is commonly a mixture of ethoxylated fatty alcohols (e.g., ceteth-20), and so on. The emulsion must be aesthetically acceptable both from visual and tactile perspective and must be stable, ensuring the stability of the entire formula, sunscreens included, to pass the requirements for expiration-date testing and functional delivery of the claimed SPF. It is not unusual to try multiple emulsions and blends to develop an acceptable formula that remains stable with the sunscreens incorporated.

Both pump sprays and pressurized aerosol sprays have similar base formulas, the difference being the use of the propellants in the pressurized aerosol forms. These forms are usually hydro-alcoholic solutions of silicones (e.g., dimethicone, cyclopentasiloxane), solvents/conditioners (e.g., glycerin), and other materials to assist in the dispensing of the sunscreens and provide aesthetically pleasing skin feel and uniform spreading of the sunscreen when applied. Propellants employed in the pressurized aerosol sprays include butane, isobutane, propane, and hydrofluorocarbon 152a, for VOC regulation.

Self-Tanning Lotions

During the late 90s and after, self-tanning lotion/sprays became popular. These formulas all rely on the chemical dihydroxy acetone (1,3 –hydrox-2-propanone). DHA reacts with the proteins in the skin to form a brown color approximately 1–2 hours after application. The concentration of the DHA (2–12%) dictates the darkness of the tan. The resultant “tan” is a purely visual, cosmetic effect, providing no UV protection to the skin as does the natural formation of melanin in an unaided exposure to sun. However, the development of a “tan” is accomplished without exposure to the other harmful effects of UVA and UVB radiation.

DHA can be formulated into creams/lotions (oil-in-water) emulsions and sprays (nonpressurized and pressurized). Formulas for these forms are similar to formulas already discussed in Hand and Body Lotions and Sunscreens. The aesthetics of the cream/lotion, the skin feel during and after application, and the development of the desired shade are the issues of importance to the formulator. Incorporation of erythrulose in the formula can impart depth and richness to the final shade obtained.

PART 6.4

ANTIPERSPIRANTS / DEODORANTS

Author

Charles Warren

The most significant difference between these two subcategories is that an A/P is an over-the-counter drug while a deodorant is purely a cosmetic product. While the formulations may be very similar in nature, the OTC drug requirements are significantly different.

Both of these product subcategories are found in similar forms. The most common forms are: stick, pressurized aerosol spray, liquid/lotion/cream, roll-on, and powder spray. These forms also come under the regulation of maximum allowable VOCs, which can vary from state to state. Prior to initiating formulation, regulatory or legal groups should be consulted regarding the applicable regulations that will impact the final formula.

Perspiration is the body's natural mechanism for cooling. Sweat, particularly in the armpit area, pools and allows bacteria to grow (warm, moist, undisturbed area). This accumulation of bacteria leads to the characteristic negative odor associated with the sweat. Deodorants are applied to allow the body to sweat but mask the unpleasant odor. Some deodorants contain materials to actually kill the bacteria while making the malodor. Antiperspirants contain materials that actually stop the sweat from exuding from the pores by creating small, gel-like plugs. These products also provide masking for any malodors that may develop from low levels of sweat that manage to exude. Because the function of the antiperspirant is to interfere or interact with a bodily function, it falls under the purveyance of an over-the-counter drug (OTC) and is bound by the specific monograph related to antiperspirants. The monograph indicates which active ingredients are allowed, what levels they may be used at, claims that may be made, etc. General OTC requirements govern stability testing required, manufacturing site registration, labeling requirements, etc. Again, of formulating OTC products, consultation with regulatory/legal groups is highly recommended.

The most common active ingredients found for the OTC products are aluminum zirconium tetrachlorohydrate (commonly used in sticks) and aluminum chlorohydrate (commonly used in sprays and roll-ons).

The base formulations for sticks generally include ingredients such as cyclopentasiloxane, stearyl alcohol, dimethicone, talc, and hydrogenated castor oil. There are a large number of other ingredients that can be used to provide different variations of stick composition. Sprays generally contain ingredients such as cyclopentasiloxane, isopropyl myristate, dimethicones, and propellants such as propane/butane/isoubutane blends and hydrofluorocarbon 152a (for VOC compliance). Lotions and creams are generally oil-in-water emulsions that contain lipoidal materials such as stearyl alcohol and ethoxylated fatty alcohols as emulsifiers.

PART 6.5

ACNE, OILY, AND AGING SKIN PRODUCT FORMULATION ESTHETIC MANAGEMENT OF ACNE-PRONE AND CLOG-PRONE SKIN

Author

Mark Lees, Ph.D., M.S., CIDESCO Diplomate

ABSTRACT

Acne and acne-prone skin conditions are frequently seen by estheticians in the salon, spa, and clinical settings. Clients who have acne-prone skin have often experienced conditions due to the use of some skin care products or cosmetics, which may contain ingredients that worsen or aggravate acne conditions or cause the development of comedones, which are follicular plugs of keratin and sebum. Comedogenic ingredients are agents that can cause or exacerbate follicular hyperkeratosis, a thickening of the walls of the follicle due to retention of keratinocytes, resulting in comedo formation. Still other ingredients can be inflammatory, causing irritation or inflammation in the follicles, which can result in sudden flares of papules or pustules. These are known as acnegenic reactions.

Successful management of acne-prone and clog-prone skin involves a number of approaches. These include: proper management of excess sebum and follicular exfoliation to loosen plugged follicles and prevent further plugging of the follicles, and the use of products that do not contain comedogenic or acnegenic ingredients, and have been documented non-comedogenic and non-acnegenic by independent testing laboratories using scientifically accepted protocols. Use-testing the products on individuals with acne-prone skin to ensure that the products meet the beauty needs of these individuals while not causing comedogenic or acnegenic reactions will lead marketers and formulators to new and effective products. This chapter includes some of these approaches with the intention of supporting formulators to create new and enhanced performing products in this category.

TABLE OF CONTENTS

6.5.1 INTRODUCTION

a. The Acne-Prone and Clog-Prone Skin: A Client Profile

The American Academy of Dermatology estimates that 40 to 50 million Americans are affected by acne and that 85% of the population has problems with acne at some time in their lives. While acne is often thought to primarily affect teenagers, it also affects many people in their adult years as well.

Estheticians frequently treat these consumers who have routine issues with acne breakouts, clogged pores, and frequent blemishes. The age of these acne-prone clients begins in the early teens and can easily reach into the 50s and sometimes even into the 60s. While acne as a condition is largely genetic and hormonal in nature, it is also influenced by the environment, including use of skin care and cosmetic products. Some skin care and cosmetic ingredients and products can increase the development of clogged pores as well as flares of acne blemishes.

Acne-prone and clog-prone skin can also be affected by aging skin conditions. The onset of wrinkles, discolorations, and elastosis associated with aging or photo-aging (aging symptoms associated with cumulative sun exposure) are a real concern for these consumers.

Many skin care products intended to help diminish the appearance of aging are also designed for helping dry skin that needs additional emollient to protect against dehydration and trans-epidermal water loss. Such materials also reduce the appearance of wrinkles and the rougher skin texture associated with dehydrated skin. These moisturizing products can be very helpful for dry and aging skin. However, because of their high emollient content, they can potentially cause problems for those clients with oily and acne-prone aging skin.

Product systems for acne-prone aging skin should contain performance ingredients that address the appearance of aging, but should be carefully formulated—avoiding ingredients known to cause clogged follicles (pores), as well as flares of acne blemishes. Professional skin care practitioners tend to attract these acne-prone aging clients because they seek professional help in treating their skin, which is both acne-prone and aging. Clinical estheticians are often charged with designing specific home care and in-clinic programs to help these clients clear their acne problems while still addressing the appearance of aging skin.

6.5.2 REVIEW OF FACTORS IN ACNE DEVELOPMENT

a. Genetics

Acne is a disorder of the skin in which the sebaceous follicle becomes obstructed by a buildup of keratinized cells mixed with excessive sebum. There are several different types of acne lesions. These include noninflammatory open comedones (blackheads) and closed comedones (whiteheads), as well as inflammatory papules and pustules. In some individuals, infected follicles can eventually develop into nodules or cysts, which can result in damage to tissue causing scarring.

The tendency to develop acne and clogged pores is largely genetic. In fact, it has been estimated that causation factors in acne is 80% genetically based. Careful management of conditions caused by these genetic factors can result in clearer skin for these acne-prone individuals.

People with acne-prone skin have two specific genetic traits. The first trait is the tendency for keratinized cells with sebaceous follicles not to shed as normal keratinocytes do; rather, they "build up" on the walls inside the follicle. This condition is known as retention hyperkeratosis.

The second genetic trait that exists in acne-prone individuals is the overproduction of sebum by the sebaceous glands. The sebum "coats over" the keratinized cell buildup on the follicle walls and adds further to the thickening of the follicle wall. Sebum also can fill the follicle and harden, thereby forming a sebaceous plug. The amount of sebum produced, the size of the sebaceous glands, and the numbers of sebaceous glands are all genetically sourced factors. It has been shown that an increased amount of sebum in the skin is directly correlated with the severity of an individual's acne condition. Therefore, it is apparent that controlling excessive sebum plays a major role in managing acne-prone skin.

Propionibacterium acnes (p. acnes) are anaerobic bacteria that exist within the flora of the sebaceous follicle. When the follicles become blocked with these plugs of hyperkeratinized cells and solidified sebum, an anaerobic environment is the result. This environment is an ideal setting for the undesirable proliferation of the p. acnes bacteria.

The sebum within the sebaceous follicles serves as the source of nourishment for p. acnes bacteria. The p. acnes bacteria produce an enzyme called lipase, which breaks triglycerides in the sebum into glycerol and fatty acids. The bacteria ingest the glycerol, and the fatty acids become a source of inflammation inside the follicle. This inflammation causes swelling in the already-occluded follicle, and can eventually cause a rupture of the follicle wall.

b. The Development of Acne Lesions

As retention hyperkeratosis occurs within the sebaceous follicle and thickens the follicle walls, the abundance of sebum coats the buildup and fills the follicle. Under these conditions, one of several types of acne lesions can develop:

A microcomedo (comedones-plural) is characterized by a "clumping" of dead cells and sebum occurring deep in a sebaceous follicle. This lesion is not visible to the naked eye and is detectable only through skin biopsies. A microcomedo is the beginning of an acne lesion. In clients with acne, there are always large numbers of unseen microcomedones for every visible lesion. It is imperative to treat these pre-lesions in order to prevent them from evolving into larger visible lesions. In the next section, we will discuss this type of treatment.

An open comedo, better known as a blackhead, is a follicle filled with dead keratinocytes and hardened sebum. The black top of an open comedo is caused by melanin pigment, likely produced as an inflammatory response. The ostium (opening; plural-ostia) of the follicle is stretched out by the debris in the follicle, hence the term open comedo. The open comedo seldom evolves into any other type of acne lesion, as the follicle is enlarged enough that oxygen is able to reach the bottom of the follicle, thereby keeping p. acnes bacteria from proliferating.

A closed comedo, sometimes called a whitehead, appears as a small bump just under the skin surface and may be viewed as a "buried" clogged follicle. Close inspection of the closed comedo reveals a very small follicle opening. In closed comedones, the follicles have filled with sebum very quickly, and the ostia are not distended.

These structures have been referred to as "time bombs" because very little oxygen can penetrate these follicles, thereby allowing p. acnes bacteria to go unchecked. The p. acnes bacteria break down the abundant sebum trapped in the follicle and produce inflammatory fatty acids. The pressure within the follicle builds until a rupture occurs in the lower walls of the follicle. This rupture causes an inflammatory immune response, with leukocytes (white blood cells) arriving at the rupture via the blood stream. Blood engulfs the follicle to allow the leukocytes to fight the bacteria. When the blood engulfs the follicle, the lesion turns red from the blood. Red lesions are indicative of immune system involvement and are known as inflammatory acne lesions. Inflammatory acne lesions include papules—red, headless, elevated lesions, often sore to the touch due to pressure within the lesions. Papules often become pustules, which are red lesions with a pustular head. Pus is comprised primarily of dead white blood cells. Open and closed comedones do not have ruptures in the follicles and are called noninflammatory acne lesions.

c. Hormonal Factors

Hormones play an extremely strong role in acne development. Male hormones known as androgens are responsible for stimulation of the sebaceous glands, which in turn produce sebum. Androgens are produced in the testes of men, and primarily in the adrenal glands in women. Androgen hormones include testosterone, androstanedione, and dihydroepiandrosterone (DHEA). The latter two androgens can bio-convert to testosterone. Testosterone is converted to the more potent dihydrotestosterone in the skin by the enzyme 5-alpha reductase.

It is dihydrotestosterone that stimulates the sebocytes, the cells within the sebaceous gland that produce sebum. As the sebocytes produce sebum, they fill with the sebum, and then rupture, spilling the sebum into the follicle.

With the onset of puberty, androgens begin being produced in both sexes. This is the time when acne first appears, in those young individuals who are genetically predisposed. Males are more likely to have acne than females in their pubescent years. Women are much more likely to have acne as adults, often never having acne flares until they are in their early 20s, or even later. Birth control, hormonal disorders, fluctuations during the menstrual cycle, pregnancy, and other hormonal issues can cause surges of androgens that can flare acne.

At menopause, estrogen levels decrease substantially. This change can result in larger concentrations of blood androgen, which can flare acne, as well as cause hirsutism (unwanted hair growth). Because estrogen is involved in the synthesis of collagen, these hormonal changes can also result in hormonally related aging skin symptoms, characterized by worsening in skin wrinkling, increased elastosis, and also may be the cause of hyperpigmentation issues or melasma.

The body responds to stress by producing cortisol in the adrenal glands. In women, most androgen is also produced in the adrenal gland. When stress is present in women, androgens may be also overproduced along with the production of cortisol. In short, stress causes hormonal fluctuations that can potentially worsen or cause acne flares.

d. Topical and Environmental Factors

We have already discussed the genetic and hormonal factors affecting the development of acne. There are also external environmental factors that can affect acne. These may include heat and UV light (sun) exposure, skin exposure to greasy or inflammatory materials, and mechanical factors such as friction from headgear or headbands.

Decades ago, dermatologists observed that a significant percentage of acne patients who wore makeup regularly seemed to have more problems with comedones and acne flares. In the 1970s, research began on comedogenicity, the tendency of cosmetic products or ingredients to cause or worsen the development of comedones, which can lead to inflammatory acne lesions. The well-known dermatologist and researcher Albert Kligman, M.D., Ph.D. coined the term "acne cosmetica," to describe this condition.

Researchers developed testing techniques to determine the severity of potential comedogenicity in both raw ingredients and finished products.

Skin care products or cosmetics that are not specifically designed for acne-prone skin can potentially cause or worsen development of comedones and cause acne flares. Skin creams, foundations, and other products that are formulated with fatty materials such as certain oils, fatty acids, or fatty esters can cause problems in acne-prone and clog-prone clients. These fatty materials can increase hyperkeratosis and plugging of the follicles and noninflammatory comedones, which may evolve into flares of inflammatory acne lesions.

Topical agents that cause or worsen the development of comedones are referred to as comedogenic. Comedones that develop from use of comedogenic products can take weeks, if not months, to appear. Non-comedogenic products are developed avoiding known comedogenic ingredients, and then tested by an independent laboratory to confirm the product's non-comedogenic status.

Sometimes products or ingredients can cause sudden flares of acne papules and pustules, but may not necessarily cause comedones to form. These materials are known as acnegenic. In acnegenic reactions, the follicle walls become irritated and inflamed from exposure to the material, resulting in sudden flares of inflammatory acne blemishes. Acnegenic reactions occur within a few days of beginning to use a new product. Acnegenic reactions have been associated with some surfactants/emulsifiers, some fragrances or essential oils, and extreme pH levels, as well as physical/mechanical contact.

Tests to determine comedogenicity are performed using both animal (rabbit ear) and human testing. Either neat ingredients or finished products can be tested. After routine exposure to the material being tested, skin is carefully checked for clinically visible comedo development, and follicular biopsies are taken to measure increases in thickness of the keratinized cell buildup on the follicle walls. These results are then compared to measurements taken in untreated skin in the same model. The measurements are then scored on a 0–3 or a 0–5 scale based on the increase of thickness measured. A score of 0 indicates no potential for comedogenicity, and as the score increases, so does the potential for comedogenicity. (See Table 1.)

Common Comedogenic Ingredients			
Highly Comedogenic (4-5/5 or 5/3)	**Moderately Comedogenic (3-4/5 or 2/3)**	**Mildly Comedogenic (2-3/5 or 1/3)**	**Noncomedogenic**
Acetylated Lanolin	Butyl Stearate	Avocado Oil	Allantoin
Coal Tar	Decyl Oleate	Caprylic/Capric	Behenic Acid
Cocoa Butter	Grape Seed Oil	Triglycerides	Butylene Glycol
Coconut Oil	Isostearyl	Corn Oil	Carbomer
Isopropyl	Neopentanoate	Evening	Castor Oil
Isostearate	Lauric Acid	Primrose Oil	Cetyl Palmitate
Isopropyl	Mink Oil	Glyceryl	Cholesterol
Linoleate	Most D & C	Stearate	Cyclomethicone
Isopropyl	Red Pigments	Hexylene	Cyclopentasiloxane
Myristate	Myristyl	Glycol	Dimethicone
Isopropyl	Lactate	Lanolin	Glycerin
Palmitate	Octyl	Lanolin Alcohol	Iron Oxides
Isostearic Acid	Palmitate	Lauryl Alcohol	Isopropyl Alcohol
Lanolic Acid	Octyldodecanol	Mineral Oil	Jojoba Oil
Linseed Oil	Sorbitan Oleate	Olive Oil	Kaolin
Myreth 3	Soybean Oil	Peanut Oil	Lecithin
Myristate	Tocopherol	Sesame Oil	Octyldodecyl Stearate
Myristyl		Safflower Oil	Octyldodecyl Stearoyl
Myristate		Stearic Acid	Stearate
Oleic Acid		Sunflower Oil	Octinoxate
Oleth-3		(Please note that	Octisalate
Oleyl Alcohol		mildly	Oxybenzone
Squalene		comedogenic	Panthenol

Common Comedogenic Ingredients			
Highly Comedogenic (4-5/5 or 5/3)	**Moderately Comedogenic (3-4/5 or 2/3)**	**Mildly Comedogenic (2-3/5 or 1/3)**	**Noncomedogenic**
		ingredients are generally not a problem when used in diluted concentrations. Check to see their ranking of concentration on the ingredient label.)	Petrolatum Phenyl Trimethicone Polysorbates Propylene Glycol Propylene Glycol Dicaprate/Dicaprylate SD Alcohol Sodium Hyaluronate Sodium PCA Sorbitol Soya Sterol Squalane Tridecyl Stearate Tridecyl Trimellitate Water Zinc Oxide Zinc Stearate

References 3,4,5,6,7

Tests are also conducted for follicle irritancy to determine acnegenicity potential. These tests may detect inflammation through follicle biopsies, or observation of flares of acne in actual product use studies.

In 1989, the American Academy of Dermatology held an invitational symposium on comedogenicity. This meeting resulted in a published report defining comedogenicity and acnegenicity, and reviewing accepted testing methods for determining comedogenic or acnegenic status of ingredients or products. One of the primary points of this report was the importance of testing the finished product. (1)

Because oils, waxes, and emollient fatty materials are primarily used in the formulation of a product vehicle, the ingredients of the product vehicle are most often the reason products are comedogenic. Performance-enhancing actives such as peptides, alpha hydroxy acids, sunscreen actives, and antioxidants are rarely comedogenic. Because the aforementioned fatty materials are often used as the vehicle in skin care products, they are used in larger concentrations and make up a significant portion of the product.

Since estheticians treat the skin solely from a topical perspective, helping consumers choose appropriate non-comedogenic and non-acnegenic products, especially for use at home, the above-stated knowledge is of great value in achieving a successful outcome.

6.5.3 MANAGEMENT OF ACNE-PRONE SKIN

There are three basic concepts in topical esthetic management of acne-prone and clog-prone skin:

a. Sebum/Oiliness Management

There is a correlation between excessive sebum and the severity of acne conditions. (2) Programs for managing acne-prone skin should include appropriate cleansers to rid the skin of excessive sebum, and help control oiliness and shininess. This is primarily achieved through surfactant cleansers that help to remove excess oil. Surfactant cleansers are user-friendly and should be developed to rinse easily. Estheticians carefully select cleansers with the appropriate amount of surfactant so they effectively cleanse the skin without overdrying it, or causing irritation from barrier function disruption. Cleansing milks are often used for makeup removal, but should be designed to not leave residues of potentially comedogenic fats on the skin. Toners for acne-prone skin sometimes contain alcohols, but overuse of these can cause dryness and potential irritation that consumers find objectionable, especially when they may be using drying agents or keratolytics to clear the acne. The main functions of toners are to remove residue from the cleanser, and to adjust the pH of the skin surface to 5.5–6.2.

Consumers with oily, clogged, or acne-prone skin generally prefer extremely lightweight moisturizers and other products such as sunscreens, foundation, or serums. Avoidance of oily materials in all wearable products helps to decrease physical oiliness, as well as likely reducing potential comedogenicity.

b. Follicular Keratolytics

Follicular keratolytic nonprescription products such as those containing alpha hydroxy acids, salicylic acid, or benzoyl peroxide help to flush follicles of debris, drying up acne lesions, breaking loose existing comedones, and chemically sloughing the follicles to help prevent development of new comedones.

Choice of active agent/ingredients and product type such as gel, liquid, or lotion, will vary with the severity of the acne condition. Aging changes and sensitive skin conditions are also a consideration. Stronger concentrations of keratolytics and antibacterials such as benzoyl peroxide or salicylic acid may be needed for more severe cases. Likewise, a vehicle containing a significant amount of SD alcohol may be helpful for a younger oily skin, but a silicone vehicle would be a better choice for an older, aging, acne-prone skin because it is less likely to dehydrate skin and accentuate wrinkles or other aging distortions.

Alpha and beta hydroxy acids are a great choice for acne-prone aging skin because they not only help to clear follicles, but they also exfoliate the surface and can significantly improve the appearance of wrinkles, hyperpigmentation, and texture issues associated with photoaging.

Benzoyl peroxide gel is often used in teenagers as well as clients of any age with more inflamed and pustular acne due to its keratolytic and antibacterial properties.

c. Avoidance of Acnegenic and Comedogenic Products

As discussed previously, treating the acne-prone and clog-prone skin with products that have been tested and determined to be non-comedogenic and acnegenic is a mainstay of esthetic management of this skin type. Moisturizers, makeup products, sunscreens, and other wearable products should all be non-comedogenic and non-acnegenic.

Vehicle and emollient ingredients are the most likely to cause comedogenicity issues and must be carefully selected. The concentration of these ingredients should also be carefully determined since the skin type is already oily. Most wearable products for this skin type are in lotion or fluid form due to their low emollient or fatty material content.

Finished products for acne-prone skin should be lightweight, as clients with oilier skin generally do not like wearing heavier or oily products.

Products must be efficacious and meet the beauty needs of the client. They must be practical and of high quality and cosmetic elegance. For example, a moisturizer that is documented non-comedogenic is of no value if it is sticky, hard to apply, or pills under makeup.

A product that is easy to use will result in better compliance with the skin care program. This will include feel and practicality, ease of application, rinsability of cleansers, and the proper selection of a container that facilitates easy application of the product. Compliance with the program will result in better results and consistency in product use.

All skin care and cosmetic products in a regimen designed for acne-prone and clog-prone skin must be documented non-comedogenic in independent testing.

6.5.4 A PROGRAM APPROACH

Education of the client with acne or clogged-pore tendency is highly important to achieve success in improving this skin condition. Estheticians will thoroughly consult with clients with acne on the client's first visit to the esthetics salon or clinic. The client should be informed as to the probable causes of the condition, the reasons for using the selected product system at home, and the need to be consistent in treating the skin to achieve positive results.

It should also be emphasized that treating any skin condition, especially acne-prone skin, involves numerous factors in both causation and treatment, and that a "program approach" is the best way to successfully improve the skin's condition. This includes using the step-by-step program as designed by esthetician, avoiding the use of potentially comedogenic products outside the program, and complying with the system instructions.

a. Case Studies

Case#1 (See Figures 1 a & 1 b.)

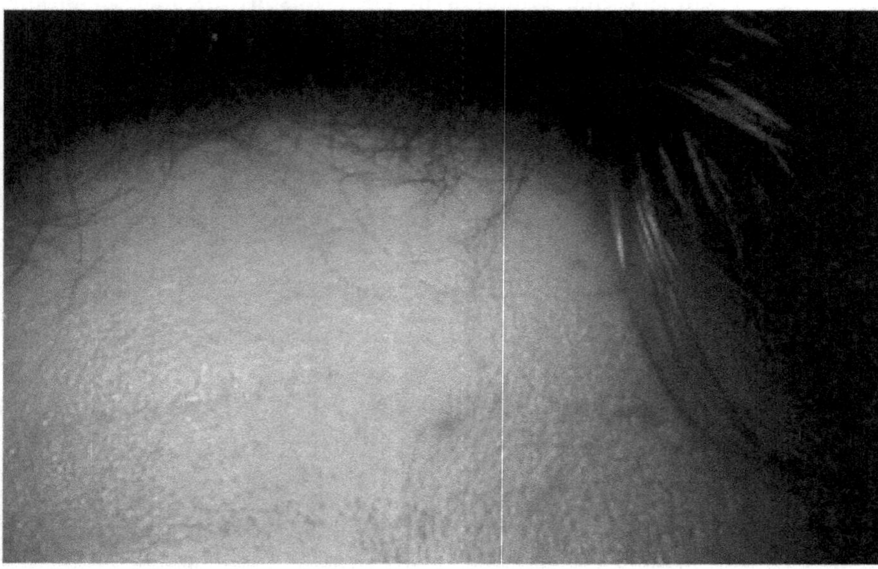

Figure 1a. Before: This skin is both clogged and dehydrated. Note the clogged follicles and obvious rough textures and uneven pigmentation.

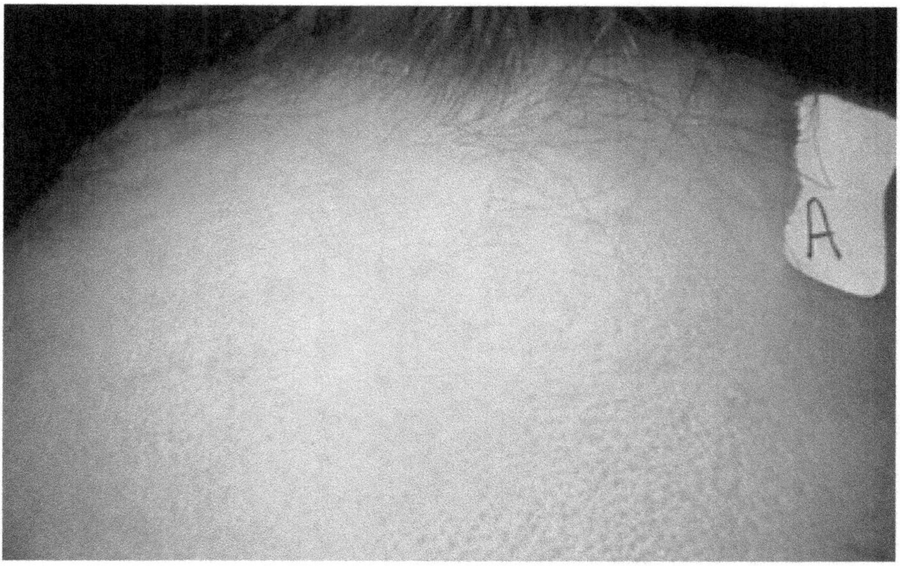

Figure b. After: After treating the skin for six weeks with a custom-designed home care program, note improvements in the clogged follicles, skin texture, hydration, clarity, and evenness of color.

(Morning)

Step 1. Skin is cleansed with a foaming rinse-off cleanser.

Step 2. A nonalcoholic toner is sprayed onto the skin and the skin is patted dry.

Step 3. Application of a 10% blended alpha and beta hydroxy acid gel-liquid

Step 4. Application of a non-comedogenic hydrating broad-spectrum sunscreen SPF-15

(Evening)

Step 1. The skin is thoroughly cleansed with non-comedogenic cleansing milk, removing all makeup.

Step 2. A nonalcoholic toner is sprayed onto the skin and the skin is patted dry.

Step 3. Application of a 10% blended alpha and beta hydroxy acid gel-liquid

Step 4. Application of a non-comedogenic hydration fluid

Cases 2–4 (See photo #2a & 2b, 3a &3b, 4a & 4b.)

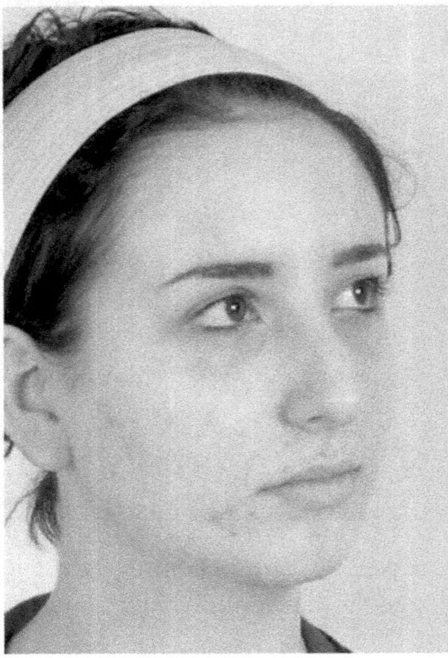

Figure 2a.

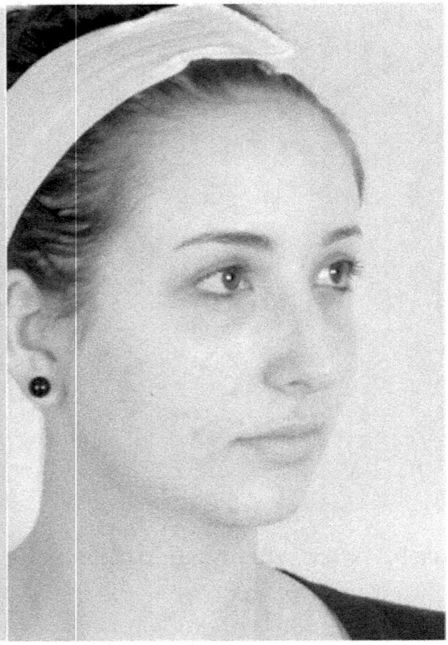

Figure 2b.

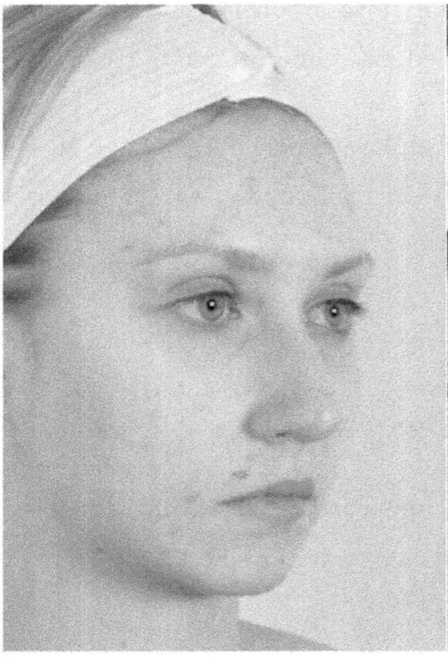

Figure 3a.

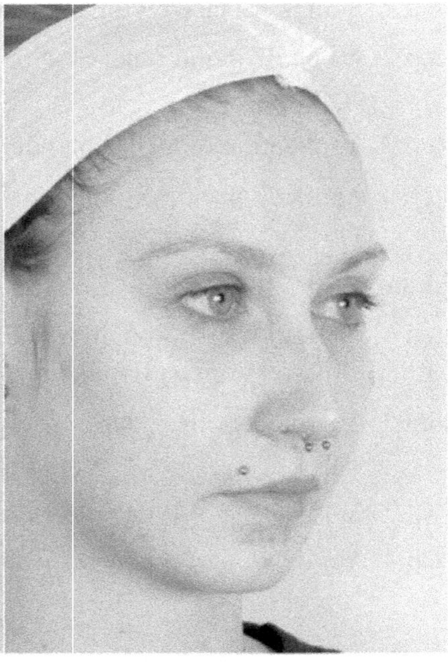

Figure 3b.

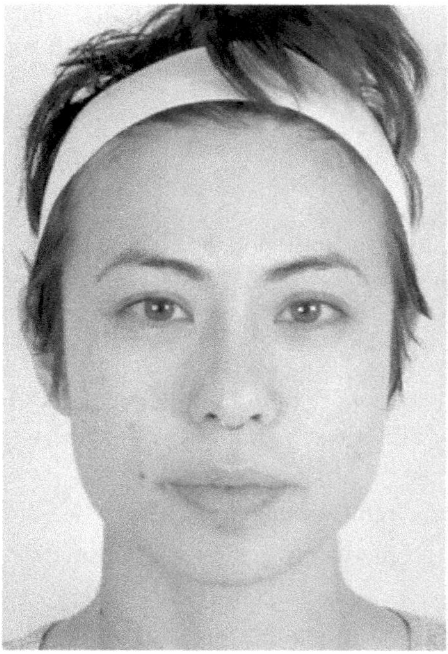

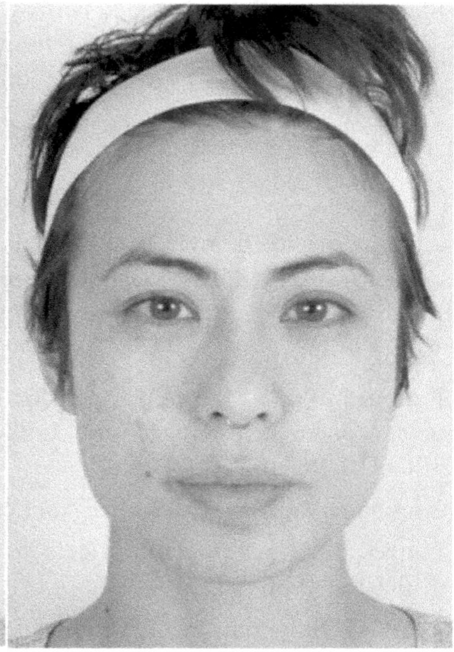

Figure 4a. **Figure 4b.**

All of these participants had both acne-prone and clog-prone skin with both non-inflammatory and inflammatory acne lesions. After four months using an esthetician-designed home care system, tremendous improvement was seen in skin clarity, tone, texture, and frequency and severity of all types of acne lesions.

Program for these case studies included:

(Morning)

Step 1. Skin is cleansed with a rinse-off foaming cleansing wash with 2.5% benzoyl peroxide (OTC).

Step 2. A toner is applied to the skin with a dampened cotton pledget and allowed to dry.

Step 3. Application of a 10% blended alpha and beta hydroxy acid gel-liquid

Step 4. Application of a non-comedogenic broad-spectrum sunscreen SPF-30

(Evening)

Step 1. The skin is thoroughly cleansed with non-comedogenic cleansing milk, removing all makeup.

Step 2. A toner is applied to the skin with a dampened cotton pledget and allowed to dry.

Step 3. Application of a 2.5% benzoyl peroxide gel medication (OTC) lightly to all areas (except eyes). Individual blemishes also treated with small additional drops of medication.

Step 4. Application of a non-comedogenic hydration fluid

REFERENCES

1. American Academy of Dermatology. Invitational symposium on comedogenicity. J. Am. Acad. Of Dermatol. 1989; 2: 272–276
2. Plewig, G. & Kligman, A. Acne and rosacea, 3rd Edition. Berlin: Springer-Verlag (2000)
3. Fulton, J., Pay, S., Fulton, J. III. Comedogenicity of current therapeutic products, cosmetics, and ingredients in the rabbit ear. J. Am. Acad. Of Dermatol. 1984; 10: 96–105
4. Kligman, A., Mills, O. Acne cosmetica. Arch Dermatol 1972; 106: 843–850
5. Lanzet, M. Comedogenic effects of cosmetic raw materials. Cosmetics & Toiletries. 1986; 101: 63–72
6. Lees, M. Skin care beyond the basics, 4th Edition. Clifton Park NY: Milady (2012) Lees, M. Unpublished data from independent comedogenicity assa

FACE AND BODY - MASKS / SCRUBS

Author

Charles Warren

As the face is an area of the body that is visible virtually all of the time, it requires formulations that function effectively and safely, leaving the consumer satisfied that the appearance and texture of the facial skin is acceptable to her/him and to the external world. Products should not create or exacerbate problems for the consumer. As facial skin is usually more sensitive than other skin on the body, formulations that would effectively clean/moisturize body skin would not be applicable to the face.

The facial skin care category is usually broken down into subcategories based on the skin type: normal, oily, sensitive, blemish control, etc. Each of these subcategories has specifically targeted products and forms. The formulator has to have a clear definition of the skin type and claims for the particular product in order to develop an effective, functional, and safe product. The products intended for blemish control or other nonstandard skin conditions are covered by OTC drug monographs and require specific active ingredients and levels, testing, manufacturing, and claims.

6.6.1 CLEANSERS/SCRUBS

As with other cleansing products, the function of facial cleansers and scrubs is to emulsify and remove excess oils and particulate from the skin. Residual makeup, flaky dry skin cells, surface bacteria, and so on must also be removed from the face. Formulas exist for normal skin, oily skin, sensitive skin, and problem (e.g., blemishes) skin.

In general, facial cleansers are an aqueous solution of surfactants and modifiers. The primary surfactants vary from soaps (e.g., ammonium stearate) to standard detergents (e.g., lauryl/laureth sulfates) to milder surfactants (e.g., taurates, sultaines). Additionally, these formulas are usually blends of surfactants such as disodium lauroamphodiacetate, sodium lauroyl (or myristoyl or cocoyl) sarcosinates, decyl or lauryl glucosides or betaines as secondary surfactants. The formulas can also contain foam boosters and modifiers to provide pleasant skin feel while washing and pleasant feel after completion (e.g., glycerin). Formulas must contain a microbiological preservative system and usually contain claims ingredients (e.g., vitamins). Low levels of fragrance are often incorporated, but fragrance-free facial cleansers are common and often desired by consumers with self-diagnosed sensitive skin. Oil-free cleansers are also available that require selections of ingredients not chemically defined as oils.

Scrubs are cleanser formulations that also include a solid particulate to assist in the mechanical abrasion and removal of the dead skin cells at the surface. These abrasive materials include: finely ground nut shells, fatty ester beads (e.g., jojoba waxes), finely ground polyethylene, etc. The choice of the abrasive material is important to ensure that the abrasion is only at the surface of the skin and does not remove the fresher skin cells below the surface. The formulations must keep the nonsoluble abrasive particulate suspended uniformly through the product for the duration of the shelf-life of the product. Suspension of the particulate can be obtained by increasing the viscosity of the system or incorporating specific polymers to aid in suspension. The surfactant systems and auxiliary ingredients are similar to those found in the cleanser formulations previously discussed.

Cleansers/scrubs for "deep cleansing" or used in "blemish" or acne control are OTC products and regulated by the monograph related to acne control. The monograph provides the allowable materials and levels that can be used as well as the claims, testing requirements, etc. for these products. In cleansers/scrubs/wipes, the most commonly used of the allowable materials is salicylic acid. This material can be incorporated in solutions of the surfactants described above for cleansers and scrubs. The formulations must be tested to ensure that the salicylic acid is stable throughout the expiration date timing indicated on the package.

6.6.2 WIPES

Facial cleansing wipes can be formulated in a dry form (i.e., wet with water prior to use) or in pre-moistened form. Pre-moistened wipes are either surfactant free, containing glycerin, propylene glycol, or other water-soluble materials or saturated with a surfactant solution. If a surfactant solution is used it would contain surfactants similar to those used in the cleansers above (i.e., disodium lauroamphodiacetate, sodium lauroyl (or myristoyl or cocoyl) sarcosinates, decyl or lauryl glucosides or betaines) used at low levels to allow ease of saturation of the nonwoven fabric and ease of use in washing the face. Wipes for acne treatment are similar solutions with the addition of one or more of the OTC-approved acne treatment ingredients (e.g., salicylic acid).

6.6.3 MOISTURIZERS

The very general subcategories for facial moisturizers are: day creams and night creams. The main difference in these two subcategories is the type and concentration of the lipoidal materials employed in the formula—lower levels of lighter moisturizers used in day creams and higher levels of heavier moisturizers used overnight.

Day creams are generally oil-in-water emulsions composed of an aqueous phase containing humectants (e.g., glycerin), lubricants/conditioners (e.g., C_{12-15} Alkyl Benzoates), polymers related to emulsion stability (e.g., carbomer), and so on, and an oil phase containing the lipoidal materials such as fatty alcohols (e.g., cetyl alcohol), mineral oil, silicones (e.g., dimethicone), lighter weight oils (e.g., isopropyl myristate), and so on. The oil phase also contains the emulsification system usually comprised of ethoxylated fatty acids (e.g., ceteth-20), higher-level PEG moieties (e.g., PEG-100 Stearate) and so on. These emulsions are formulated to be very light to the touch, spread quickly and evenly over the skin, and absorb quickly. Day creams are also available in "oil-free" formulas. These formulas usually contain lipoidal materials that are not technically oils in the lipid phase. An example would be ethylhexyl palmitate.

Many day creams also contain sunscreens to attain an SPF rating. The addition of sunscreens makes the formula an OTC drug, and all of the issues indicated in the section on sunscreens for the body are applicable. The monograph provides the allowed sunscreens and levels, testing, registrations, claims, etc.

Night creams typically contain higher levels of heavier, more efficacious occlusive agents. Applied before going to bed, the "greasiness" of these creams while sleeping is not an issue and the better occlusive materials used allow the surface skin to be hydrated from beneath. These formulations are also water-in-oil emulsions containing similar materials to the day creams but also containing higher levels of materials such as mineral oil and petrolatum. Sunscreens are rarely contained in night creams because there is no exposure to UV radiation overnight. Night creams would not be acceptable for daytime use due to the increased oiliness.

6.6.4 TREATMENTS

The area of skin treatment is very complicated. Some treatments (e.g., acne) are an OTC drug, covered by a specific monograph. Some treatments (e.g., masques) are purely cosmetic and are used on an occasional basis. In formulation in this category, the formulator needs to be careful that the desired claims do no move a purely cosmetic product into the realm of a new drug, subject to a very different set of requirements. For example, "improving the appearance of fine lines and wrinkles" is a purely cosmetic claim, while "eliminating fine lines and wrinkles" is a drug claim. The former can be accomplished by the use of alpha-hydroxy acid treatments; the latter has been reserved for medical treatments such as dermabrasion or injection. If formulating in this category, close consultation with marketing, regulatory, and legal groups is highly advisable.

Blackhead/acne treatment masks usually fall under the OTC acne treatment monograph and are bound by all of the provisions therein. Benzoyl peroxide (2–10%) and salicylic acid are the most commonly used, allowed ingredients in this product grouping. These treatments are usually paired with a salicylic acid containing cleanser or scrub as a first step in a regimen. Benzoyl peroxide or salicylic acid is then applied to the area to be treated. All of these products work by killing the acne bacteria and loosening the upper layers or agglomerations of dead skin cells in the pores and inflamed areas.

Surface fine lines and wrinkles result from the aging process and accumulated exposure to UV radiation. Cosmetic treatment of fine lines and wrinkles involves only the uppermost layer of the stratum corneum. Deep wrinkles in the skin can only be treated medically. Retinol or retinal and retynyl derivatives are the most common active ingredients in this grouping. This grouping would also include the α- and β-hydroxyl acids (e.g., glycolic acid). These active ingredients work by removing the top layers of the stratum corneum, exposing the fresher, more compact lower layers. As these uppermost layers are removed, the appearance of fine lines and wrinkles is reduced, leaving the skin looking fresher and more uniform. Because these materials work chemically to removes the skin cells, they are often referred to as "chemical peels," differentiated from the abrasive action of the scrubs containing fine particulate materials.

Masks are usually very thick water-in-oil emulsions that are intended to be applied on the face and neck, left on for a prolonged period, and then rinsed off. Many of these formulas contain kaolin, bentonite, or other clays to provide bulk and thickness and support the position of a "deep treatment."

Another grouping in facial treatments is astringents/toners. These products are usually alcoholic or hydroalcoholic solutions meant to dry and slightly tighten the skin after cleansing. "Witch Hazel" extract is a commonly found ingredient in these type formulations.

Another category of skin treatments are the skin-lightening or skin-brightening products, used to correct darker portions of the skin (lighteners) or provide a fresher, brighter appearance to the skin. Skin lighteners are covered under an OTC monograph. The only currently approved active ingredient in the U.S. monograph is hydroquinone. Other ingredients (e.g., kojic acid) are allowed in other countries. Rules and regulations around skin lightening are in a constant state of flux and require consultation with Regulatory/Legal groups prior to initiating formulation. Incorporation of a sunscreen ingredient is also required for these products in the U.S.

6.6.5 PERFUMES/FRAGRANCES

Actual perfume oils are created from individual fragrance ingredients by highly skilled and extensively trained formulators. Most perfumers work at fragrance suppliers and work with internal customer service/fragrance evaluators to develop fragrances specifically for client/customer groups. The cosmetic formulator will select and use these fragrances to formulate the consumer fragrance products that actually go to market.

Perfumes/colognes/eau de toilettes/etc. all have specific definitions related to the concentration of the fragrance oil in an alcoholic system. Body splashes and sprays are a lower level of fragrance oils in a hydroalcoholic system.

Fragrance ingredients can be skin sensitizers, and different fragrance oil ingredients become eliminated on a fairly regular basis. Perfumers, fragrance suppliers, and their internal safety and regulatory groups maintain current status on the regulatory and safety environment and are of great assistance to formulators who do not deal with this ever-changing environment on a regular basis.

PART 6.7

SHAVING PREPARATIONS: PRE AND POST

Author
Charles Warren

The removal of hair from undesired areas is another subgroup off specialty skin care products. The unwanted hair can be removed mechanically (e.g., shaving) or chemically (e.g., depilation). All of the processes are aided by various products, and all of the processes leave the skin in a state that usually requires some degree of post-process conditioning.

Oftentimes, men's and women's products in the subgroups are differentiated solely by fragrance, packaging, and advertising claims. Other products are gender focused.

6.7.1 MEN'S PRODUCTS

a. Shave Creams

Men's shave creams are available in a multitude of forms: pressurized foams, pressurized self-foaming gels, creams, soaps, liquids, etc. The pressurized foams and self-foaming gels are the largest segments. The purpose of all of these products is to help hydrate the individual hairs, raising them from the surface of the skin and making them easier to cut with a razor.

Pressurized foams are generally an aqueous solution of fatty acid soaps, formed *in situ* by combining a long-chain fatty acid (usually palmitic or stearic) with an alkali (such as triethanolamine or sodium hydroxide). In addition there will be secondary surfactants (e.g., sodium lauryl or laureth sulfate), emulsifiers, such as ethoxylated fatty alcohols (e.g., laureth-23), fragrance and, if needed, skin moisturizers (e.g., glycerin). Some foams incorporate menthol for a cooling sensation during the actual shaving process and after completion.

The soap-base is then placed in a can with a propellant system (propane, butane, isobutane, etc.). By shaking immediately before use, propellant is incorporated into the aqueous soap base and, when dispensed, expands to create the thick creamy foam.

Self-foaming gels have become extremely popular with both men and women. These products are both a result of formulation and mechanical dispensing. The gel itself is composed of a soap base, not unrelated to the based used in the creams above. Usually the gel base will include a material such as hydroxyethylcellulose to provide the gel-like form when dispensed. The gel base will also include secondary surfactants, humectants (e.g., glycerin or sorbitol), fragrances, colors, etc. The gel base is placed in a piston can and the propellant system is placed in the lower chamber to push the gel through the dispenser as the gel is dispensed. Isopentane is injected into the gel base after filling, and it is this material that causes the gel to blossom into a foam when dispensed onto the hand. This blossoming is slower than the shave cream foam generation and requires some mechanical action with the hands to develop.

As the shave creams and gels employ hydrocarbons as propellants or dispensing media, they too fall under VOC regulations. Formulating in these arenas requires consult with appropriate regulatory and legal groups to ensure necessary compliance.

Shaving lotions (nonpressurized) are generally oil-in-water emulsions that contain blends of surfactants (anionic and or nonionic), emulsifiers (e.g., ethoxylated fatty alcohols), humectants (e.g., glycerin or sorbitol), fragrances, etc. These are applied as a lotion and serve the same general purpose of hair hydration and lift for razor removal.

Simple shaving liquids can be formulated from aqueous solutions of humectants (e.g., propylene glycol or sorbitol) or a blend of lightweight oils such as isopropyl palmitate. While effective, these liquids do not enjoy the widespread popularity of the shaving creams or gels.

b. After-Shave Lotions

Both the process of shaving with a razor and the materials used (e.g., shaving cream) can leave the skin mildly abraded and/or dry. After-shave treatments (liquids and lotions) can be developed to ameliorate these effects.

The simplest after-shave is a hydroalcoholic solution of fragrance. These can also incorporate hydoalcoholic-soluble ingredients such as glycerin, sorbitol, menthol, etc., depending on the desired end product.

After-shave lotions have also become popular. In general, these are thin, oil-in-water emulsions containing an aqueous phase with water, humectants, nonionic surfactants, and other water-soluble ingredients and an oil phase containing fatty alcohols (e.g., cetyl alcohol), fatty esters (e.g., isopropypalmitate), emulsifiers (e.g., ethoxylated fatty alcohols), etc. These formulas are similar to facial moisturizers and hand and body lotions, but are balanced to be much thinner and less occlusive. Again, their purpose is to ameliorate the negative effects of shaving, immediately after the process.

6.7.2 WOMEN'S PRODUCTS

a. Shaving Products

The largest category of shaving products for women are the self-foaming shave gels, which, in base formula, are identical to the same products described for men above. They are differentiated by fragrance, concentration of conditioning agents (e.g., sorbitol), and packaging graphics. In form and function they are identical.

b. Depilatories

Depilatories are formulas that actually shear the hair off (at the skin level), chemically. They employ an alkaline solution of calcium or potassium thioglycolate—the same thioglycolate ion that is employed in permanent waving. The formulations are made alkaline (pH 9–10) with a strong alkali, such as sodium hydroxide. The base cream formulation is usually an oil-in-water emulsion consisting of a water phase containing the thioglycolate, alkali, and any other water-soluble ingredients desired, and an oil phase consisting of fatty alcohols (e.g., cetyl alcohol), oils (e.g., mineral oil, fatty esters), and the emulsification system (usually ethoxylated fatty alcohols or other fatty esters). Emulsions may also contain polymeric materials (e.g., cross-linked polymers) that are compatible with the reducing agent and the highly alkaline water phase.

Due to the reactive nature of depilatory formulations, skin irritation can be expected and, therefore, the formulator needs to include ingredients in the formula to mitigate the dryness and irritation that may result. Materials such as mineral oil, isopropyl myristate, and other fatty ester oils can be used to keep the skin soft and moisturized and reduce contact with the active ingredients.

While not chemical depilatories, other forms of depilation are available for women. These include purely mechanical hair removal (e.g., depilation mitts) to waxes, which involve placing liquefied wax on the area for depilation and removal of hardened wax (and imbedded hair) via cloth strips while affixed while wax is still in molten phase. These waxes are usually blends of rosinates (e.g., hydrogenated rosinate) and beeswax, modified with materials to control melting points and pliability.

c. Bleaches

While not technically hair-removal formulations, light bleach formulations are available for hair on the upper lip and around the mouth (e.g., chin). These products bleach the melanin in the darker hair, leaving it white or almost transparent. Because these hairs are usually fine (e.g., small diameter) the bleaching makes them less visible to the eye. The base formulas are usually oil-in-water emulsions or simple polymeric (e.g., carbomer) solutions that contain low levels (2–5%) hydrogen peroxide, as the active bleaching agent.

PIGMENTED COSMETICS

PART 6.8

COLOR COSMETICS: AN INTRODUCTION TO FORMULATION AND APPROACHES FOR MASCARAS, FOUNDATIONS AND LIPSTICKS

Authors

Germain Puccetti, Nevine Issa, and Hani Fares

ABSTRACT

The chapter will first cover the basic formulation types and important considerations in each of the categories and then take an in-depth look at the role and benefits of ingredients within these types of products and their influence on the finished formulation performance. In addition, advanced benefits such as water and wear resistances will be addressed in terms of ingredients and their influence on the formulation's behavior. Finally, the use of skin care ingredients in color cosmetics will be presented and their benefits in the formulations discussed from a formulator and from a consumer perspective.

TABLE OF CONTENTS

6.8.1 COLOR COSMETICS AND THE CONSUMER PERSPECTIVE

The use of cosmetics for beautification has been known in multiple cultures such as Egypt and China since antiquity. Color cosmetics represent a subcategory of all cosmetics, and they are defined as bringing color changes to the appearance of various parts of the consumer, whether face, neck or arms, hands, legs, and feet. This class of cosmetic products can affect the physical appearance such as eyelash shape and length, in addition to the visual perception such as darkening eyelashes and giving a more pleasing visual contrast.

Color cosmetics encompass a wide range in products targeting different physical aspects: the eye area (mascaras, eyeliners, eye shadows), facial skin (foundations, concealers, blushes), the lip area (lipsticks, lip-gloss, lip-liners), finger- and toenails (nail lacquers).

In all these areas, products often combine optical benefit (color, sparkle, diffusion) with skin appearance improvements (even toner, concealers, wrinkle fillers, and active ingredients such as firming or healthy nail growth).

6.8.2 FOUNDATIONS

Three main types of foundations can be differentiated: water based, oil based, and silicone. Foundations are intended to provide desired coverage of skin inhomogeneities as well as color shades while maintaining the skin's natural breathing.

Color shade changes can readily be adapted by slight changes in the blend of color pigments used, and consumers have a generally wide range in shades at their disposal to either maintain, enhance, or strengthen their natural skin tone. Foundations are one class of products used to counter the perceived age of a person by matching pigment composition to the type of skin imperfections of a consumer [1–3].

Skin inhomogeneities are of two types: brown/age spots and rednesses. Both need to be addressed by a foundation to provide a maximum impact on the skin's visual appearance. An example is given in Figure 26.1 below, where a sheer foundation application can be separated into both color components corresponding to respective inhomogeneities. One can clearly see that this foundation is more efficient at covering rednesses than brown spots.

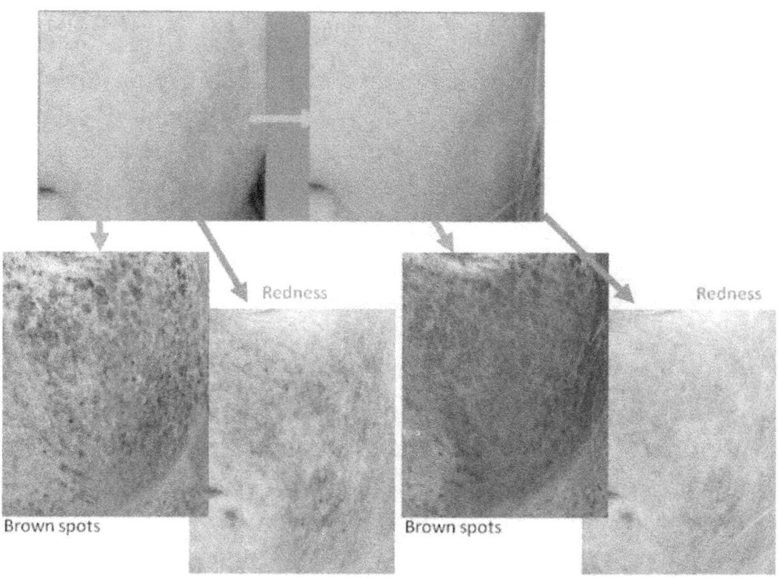

Figure 26.1. Effect of a sheer foundation on the coverage of brown/age spot and redness imperfections. Natural light images of a panelist are shown on the top: before (left) and after (right) foundation application. Both images have been filtered for their brown and red color channels to visualize respective skin imperfections and the efficiency of the formulation at covering each of these.

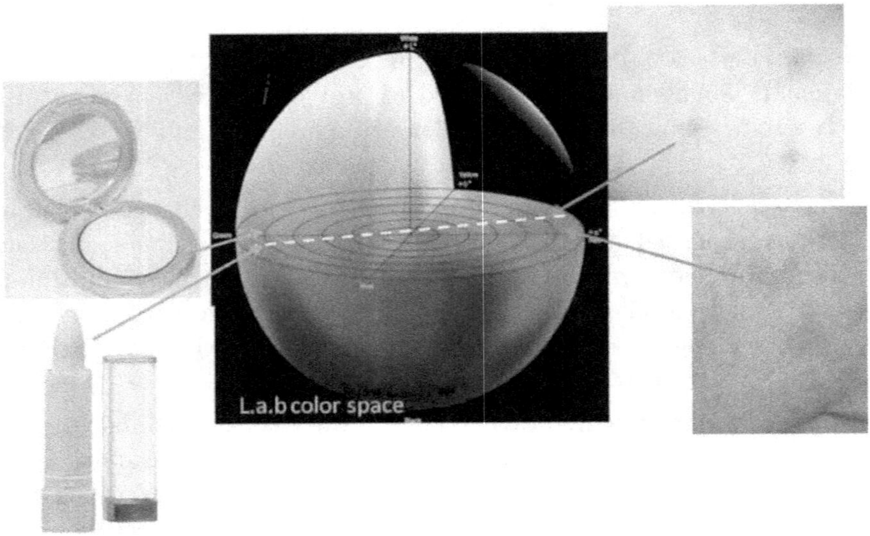

Figure 26.2. Examples of complementary color approaches used to counter skin local imperfections, e.g., insect bites, redness spots

It is therefore to add pigments countering both types of imperfections. This can be performed by two approaches: (a) adding pigments of solid mass tone or neutral fillers such as talc or titanium dioxide to give more color-neutral coverage, or (b) countering the imperfection color by means of a complementary color pigment. The last approach is commonly used in spot concealers to hide local rednesses, in which case a greenish pigment is used. Examples are shown in Figure 26.2 below.

Complementary color concealers bring selective color corrections to local areas and are more appropriate for local corrections. The final aspect should be as close as possible to the desired skin natural tone. For larger areas of skin imperfections or inducing a skin shade change, pure high-coverage cosmetic products with the intended skin color shade are more adapted.

Thirdly, foundation layer breathability is very important when applied to skin to avoid sebum and water buildup near the interface between foundation and the skin. The natural membrane property of skin needs to be maintained and disturbed as little as possible to avoid rash and more severe side effects. Film-forming ingredients such as polymers can help here while maintaining film integrity and limit rub-off. Different regions of the world such as Europe or some Asian countries will place more importance on skin compatibility and therefore avoid "heavy" (oil-based) or high coverage foundations containing high pigment loads and thus more prone to skin occlusion effects. The following foundation illustrates the approach of a more sheer "breathable" liquid foundation in which film integrity and wear resistance were brought by an acrylate/C_{12}–C_{22} alkyl methacrylate copolymer. This polymer also ensures good adhesion to the skin.

a. Formulas

Formula 26.1. Transfer resistant liquid foundation with an SPF of 23 (*in vitro* test)

Phase	Ingredients	% W/W
A	Water	50.95
	Glycerin	2
	disodium edta	0.1
	triethanolamine	0.1
	Acrylic Acid/VP crosspolymer	0.1
B	SB700 Silica Beads	1
	BTD-401 ITT Treated TIO2	5.08
	BYO-12 ITT Treated Yellow Iron Oxide	0.48
	BRO-12 ITT Treated Red Iron Oxide	0.18
	BBO-12 ITT Treated Black Iron Oxide	0.1
	O-13 ITT Treated Sericite	1.56
C	GLYCERYL Stearate (and) Laureth-23	2.3
	Ceteareth-20	1.3
	Decyl Oleate	1.5
	Isocetyl Stearate	0.75
	Octocrylene	3
	Ethylhexyl salycilate	3
	Avobenzone	2
	Dimethicone	3
	Trimethylsiloxyphenyl Dimethicone	7
	Triacontanyl PVP	3
	VP/Eicosene Copolymer	2
D	Cyclopentasiloxane	6
E	Acrylates/C12–22 Alkylmethacrylate Copolymer	2
	Caprylyl Glycol, Phenoxyethanol	1.5
	Total:	100

PROCEDURE

1. Pre-weigh water, glycerin, and disodium EDTA and mix until clear; add TEA and mix until uniform. Sprinkle ultrathix slowly until all is in. Let mix for one hour until completely hydrated.
2. Weigh ingredients of phase B and pulverize for about ten minutes.
3. In a separate beaker, add ingredients of phase C and heat to 75–80°C while mixing.
4. Switch phase C to homomixer and add phase B. Homomix phase B+C, maintaining temperature 75–80°C
5. Heat phase A to 75–80°C and add phase B+C to A while homogenizing. Homomix for about ten minutes.
6. Begin cooling the batch to 55°C. Add phase D and continue homomixing.
7. Switch to sweep agitation and cool to 35°C. Add phase D and continue mixing to R.T.

Initial viscosity: LVT-TB @ 5rpm = 7X800 = 5,600 cps PH = 6.53

24-hour viscosity: LVT-TB @ 5rpm @ 25c: 10 × 800 = 8,000 cps PH = 6.54

Formula 26.2. Silicone Foundation

Phase	INCI	% W/W
A	Ethylhexyl Palmitate	3.00
	Isodecyl Neopentanoate	4.00
B	Cyclopentasiloxane, PEG/PPG-18/18 Dimethicone	5.00
	Lauryl PEG-9, Polydimethyl Siloxyethyl Dimethicone	2.30
	Cyclopentasiloxane, Dimethicone Vinyltrimethylsiloxysilicate crosspolymer	5.00
	Cyclopentasiloxane	6.00
C	Silica	1.00
	Titanium Dioxide (and) Isopropyl Titanium Triisostearate	6.70
	Iron Oxides (and) Isopropyl Titanium Triisostearate	0.87
	Iron Oxides (and) Isopropyl Titanium Triisostearate	0.33

Phase	INCI	% W/W
C	Iron Oxides (and) Isopropyl Titanium Triisostearate	0.14
	Mica (and) Isopropyl Titanium Triisostearate	1.10
D	Water	60.31
	Sodium Chloride	0.50
E	Propylene Glycol	3.00
	Phenoxyethanol, MethylParaben, Butyl Paraben, EthylParaben, Propylparaben	0.75
	Total:	100

PROCEDURE

1. Heat phase A to 72°C until melted and uniform. Cool to RT.
2. Add phase A to phase B at RT. Mix until uniform. *No heat.*
3. Pulverize phase C ingredients and add to phase AB mixture using high-speed mixing.
4. In a separate vessel, premix phase D ingredients homogenizing for ten minutes.
5. Premix phase E ingredients until uniform.
6. Add phase E to D (premix) and mix until uniform.
7. Add phase DE to phase ABC very slowly with paddle mixing.
8. When completely mixed, switch to homogenizer and homomix for five minutes.

Viscosity: with 0.1% oatmeal: 42 × 2000 = 84,000 cps, PH = 4.94

Formula 26.3. Radiance Skin Illuminating Foundation

Phase	Ingredients	% W/W
A	Deionized Water	36.46
	Glycerin	1.00
	Disodium EDTA	0.10
	Magnesium Aluminum Silicate	1.00
	Xanthan Gum	0.20
	Butylene Glycol	4.00
B	SB700 Silica Beads	1.00
	BTD-401 ITT Treated TIO2	6.78
	BYO-12 ITT Treated	0.87

Phase	Ingredients	% W/W
B	Yellow Iron Oxide	
	BRO-12 ITT Treated	0.33
	Red Iron Oxide	
	BBO-12 ITT Treated	0.20
	Black Iron Oxide	
	O-13 ITT Treated Sericite	1.82
C	GLYCERYL Stearate (and) Behenyl Alcohol (and) Palmitic Acid (and) Stearic Acid (and) Lecithin (and) Lauryl Alcohol (and) Myristyl Alcohol (and) Cetyl Alcohol	5.00
	C12–15 Alkyl Lactate	3.00
	Decyl Oleate	1.50
	Isocetyl Stearate	0.75
	Ethylhexyl Methoxycinnamate	7.00
	Ethylhexyl Salycilate	3.00
	Dimethicone	1.00
D	Acrylates/C12–22 Alkylmethacrylate Copolymer	1.00
E	Cyclopentasiloxane	7.50
F	Diazolidinyl Urea (and) Iodopropynyl Butylcarbamate	0.50
G	Styrene/Acrylates Copolymer	10.99
H	Mica (and) Titanium Dioxide	3.00
	Total:	100

PROCEDURE

1. Heat water to 75°C, add remaining ingredients of phase A (pre-wet gums with Butylene Glycol).
2. Mix well until gums are completely hydrated.
3. Pre-blend phase B (pulverize). Add phase B to phase C at 75°C using homomixer.
4. Add phases B & C (70–75°C) to phase A (75°C) using homomixing. Homogenize for ten minutes.
5. Add phase D with homomixing; mix until uniform.
6. Cool to 55°C with slow homomixing; add phases E & F (pre-mixed). Mix until uniform. Add phase G. Mix until uniform.

7. Switch to sweep-mixing; cool batch to room temperature with sweep-mixing. Add phase H to batch; mix until uniform.

Common ingredients of a liquid foundation:

b. Pigments

Pigments impart color to the final formulation. They can be of two types: absorption pigments of interference pigments. Absorption pigments give color by absorbing part of the visible light spectrum. Their observed color results from reflection of the nonabsorbed light spectrum. Combining absorption pigments needs to consider the reflected light colors in order to avoid overlap of reflected light wavelengths and absorbed wavelengths. This is termed "subtraction color composition." It is illustrated by a trichromatic schematic showing that blue is the result of light absorption in the yellow or that red is the resulting color of light absorption at red wavelengths. Combining red and blue absorption pigments will yield a green shade instead of magenta. A good example of this color composition system is the CMY (cyan/magenta/yellow) system widespread in the printing industry. In a subtractive system, one starts from a neutral white light spectrum and each pigment removes a specific wavelength region from the white spectrum, leaving its remaining colors [4].

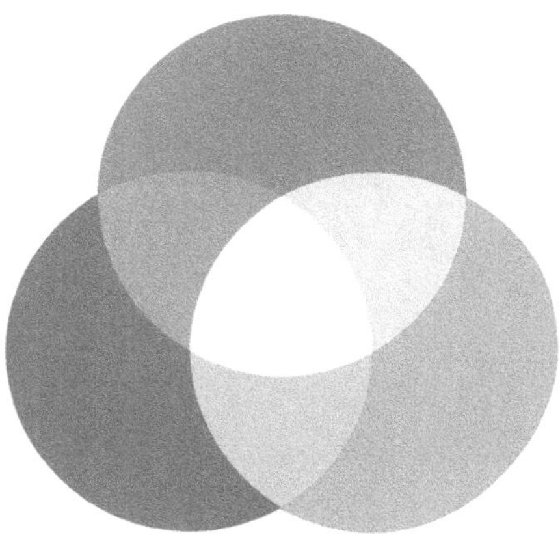

Figure 26.3. RGB and CMY trichromic color composition systems.

On the contrary, additive colors are obtained when pigments are the actual source of the color shade. Interference pigments act by selective reflection of a wavelength from the visible spectrum, and as such, pigments act similar to a light source. In this system, using a red and blue light sources will give a magenta light. In the additive composition system, one starts here with an empty light spectrum (dark). Each interference pigment adds a source of light to this dark background, which color relates to the reflective interference wavelength.

An illustration of the differences is given in Figure 26.4.

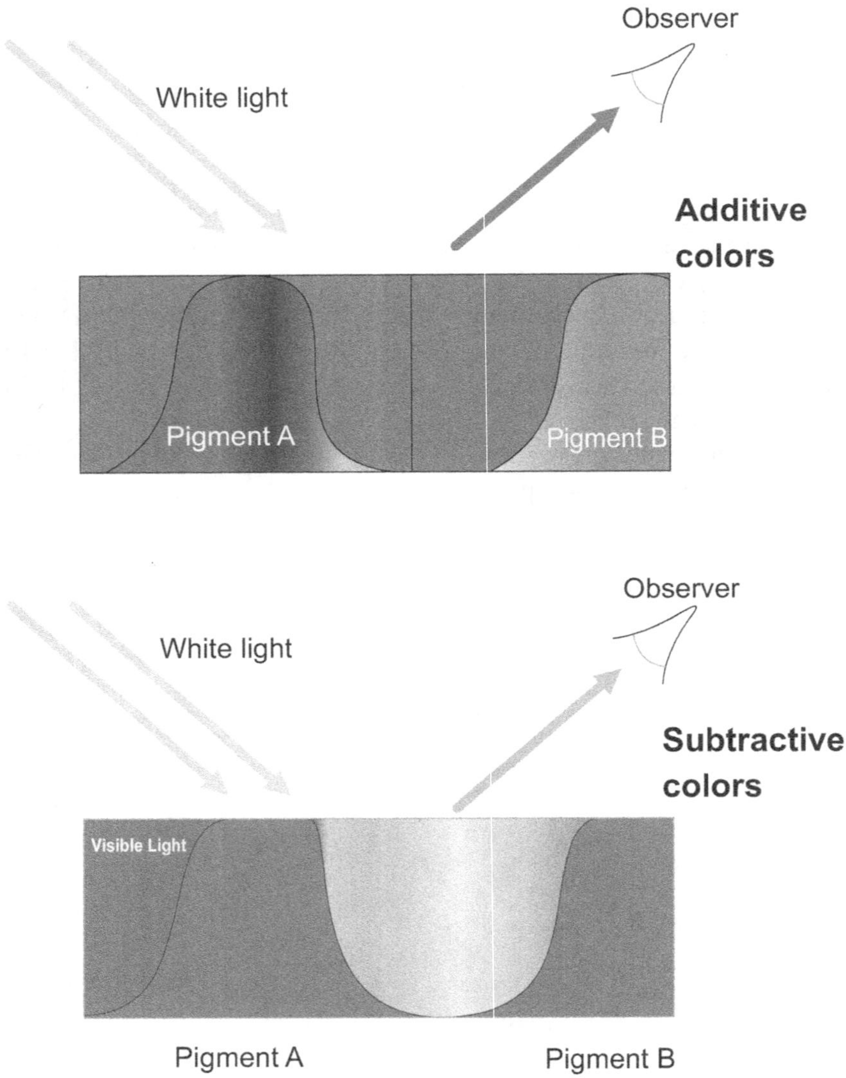

Figure 26.4. Additive (top) and subtractive (bottom) color composition systems

Fillers

The purpose of fillers is to opacify formulations to adjust the degree of transparency from a high-coverage foundation to a sheer foundation without affecting the color shade of a formulation. Fillers can lighten a formulation (higher concentrations above 5%) and they can induce a thickening of formulations. The most common fillers are titanium dioxides (white), talc (used less now), and silica particles. The particle size of fillers also influences the optical appearance of the product on skin.

Finer particles will give a softer appearance than larger particles. Finally, silicon dioxide particles are sometimes used to bring a slight light-scattering effect in foundations applied to skin, resulting in a soft-focus effect. They are often termed "light diffusion particles" and are generally coated for secondary purposes such as more hydrophilic/hydrophobic characteristics. The coating can also affect the optical refractive index and enhance the light-diffusion effect. In addition, the coating generally prevents any sensitization risks when applied to sensitive skin.

Surfactants

These ingredients are often dependent on the type and concentrations of pigments as well as fillers. Their role is to disperse and maintain a homogenous dispersion in the liquid form. Common surfactants include stearates, dimethicones, oleates, and polyoxyethylene ethers (nonionic).

Thickeners

Thickeners serve to bring more texture to the formulation while also reducing the risk of pigment sedimentation inside a bottle. They are used in low amounts when needed, since the pigments and fillers will bring a formulation quite high in viscosity.

Film formers

Oils and silicones can be used to enhance spreadability on skin. Dimethicones are typical for spreadability while giving a dryer skin feel post-application. These compounds will also help skin adhesion of the formulation during its first minute following application. A good compromise needs to be reached in terms of time of setting of the foundation on the skin and time allowed for a consumer to evenly spread a formulation over the desired area.

Polymers

Polymers are widely used in foundations for multiple reasons. They will enhance film adhesion on skin (e.g., acrylate/C_{12}–C_{22} alkylmethacrylate copolymer). Polymers also bring stability to the foundation film by maintaining pigments evenly dispersed while providing a degree of porosity and breathability (e.g., triacontanyl PVP). As mentioned before, film breathability is very important for skin to avoid occlusion effects. Several polymers are often combined to ensure adhesion on skin and good retention of pigments over time of wear. This last benefit is responsible for wear resistance of a foundation to avoid any rub-off or staining of consumer clothes during the daily wear time of a foundation. Lastly, polymers can also bring a mattifying effect via sebum absorption/trapping and thus prevent the development of skin shine and oily appearance.

Additional ingredients

In addition to water, pH adjusters, preservatives, and antioxidants fall in this category to address the stability of the final formulation and its good compatibility with skin. Alcohols can also be used to give a slightly faster drytime.

6.8.3 LIPSTICKS AND LIP-GLOSSES

The lip area of a person has been one of the attraction features of beauty in many cultures around the world [5]. Properties such as fullness, shape, definition, and volume have all been associated with desire to enhance beauty and attractiveness. An example of extreme contrast enhancement can be seen for geishas in the Japanese culture, in which case bright red lip color is commonly used on a near-white skin background makeup. It is therefore natural for consumers to have a high interest in products enhancing the lips. While in the past, lipsticks have mainly focused on bringing decorative benefits (color shade, gloss), they now also bring functional (sun protection) and skincare (moisturizing, plumping) benefits to the lip skin.

The importance of lipsticks and lip-gloss in modern culture can be seen by the wide selection in color shades available in commerce. An interesting point is the large proportion of color shade names associated with fruits or senses such as berry, pomegranate, plum, luscious, passion, sensual, all of which use the mentally associated image of fresh/richness with an enhanced feel of beauty.

a. Formulas

Formula 26.4. Example of transfer-resistant lipstick formulation

Phase	Ingredients	% W/W
A	Ozokerite	10.50
	Polyethylene	5.00
	Octyldodecyl Stearate	13.00
	Diisopropyl Adipate	2.00
	Isocetyl Stearoyl Stearate	14.70
	Shea Butter	4.00
	C_{12-15} Alkyl Lactate	11.00
	Hydrogenated Polyisobutene	5.00
	VP/Eicosene Copolymer	5.00
	VP/Hexadecene Copolymer	5.00
	Tocopheryl Acetate	0.20

Phase	Ingredients	% W/W
A	Retynyl Palmitate	0.10
B	Isopropylparaben (and) Isobutylparaben (and) Butylparaben	0.40
C	Red 7 Lake (C6507 D&C Red #7 Calcium Lake)	1.00
	Iron Oxides (C33-8073 Yellow Iron Oxide)	1.00
	Titanium Dioxide (White)	1.20
	Iron Oxides (C33-5198 Black Iron Oxide)	0.35
	Isocetyl Stearoyl Stearate	3.45
	Tricontanyl PVP	0.10
D	Mica	13.00
	Mica (and) Iron Oxides (and) Titanium Dioxide	4.00
	Total:	100

Procedure

1. Prepare phase C color grind using roller mill (Melt Ganex® WP-660; add to color mix before milling)
2. Melt phase A ingredients. Heat to 90–95°C; mix until uniform.
3. Cool batch to 82–85°C.
4. Add phase B; mix until smooth.
5. Add phase C color grind; mix approximately 30 min.
6. Add phase D, avoid aerating batch; mix until uniform.
7. Pour samples at 82–85°C.

Formula 26.5. Example of lip-gloss formulation.

Phase	Ingredients	% W/W
A	VP/Hexadecene Copolymer	20.30
	Polybutene	19.00
	Isostearyl Neopentanoate	8.20
	Ethylhexyl Palmitate	8.00
	Octyldodecyl Stearate	8.00

Phase	Ingredients	% W/W
A	Myristyl Lactate	9.00
	Tribehenin	3.00
	Beeswax	3.00
	Tocopheryl Acetate	0.10
B	Isopropylparaben (and) Isobutylparaben (and) Butylparaben	0.40
	Mica	11.00
	Mica (and) Titanium Dioxide (and) Red 7 Lake (and)	
	Hydrogenated Polyisobutene (and) Palmitic Acid (Cellini Red)	2.00
C	Mica (and) Iron Oxides (and) Titanium Dioxide (Gemtone Tan Opal)	8.00
	Total:	100

PROCEDURE

1. Melt phase A ingredients; heat to 85–90°C until melted and uniform.
2. Cool batch to 80°C.
3. Add phase B; mix until uniform.
4. Add phase C; avoid aerating batch; mix until uniform.
5. Pour samples at 80°C.

b. Color

First of all, lipsticks are intended to enhance or bring color to lips. This is generally achieved by adding colorants to the product, which is applied to lips as a thin coating. Most shades found nowadays contain some red dye and range from pale pink/orange to bright red and to darker tones of red, brown, or purple. Some unusual lipstick colors such as green, blue, or black can also be found. The color imparts a higher visibility to lips and shades are also considered to reflect the occasional environment of the consumer. Color has also been found in the form of skin dyes such as eosin and bromofluoresceins. These dyes penetrate slightly into the first layer of lip skin, which makes them more wear resistant. As a consequence, they also can induce some sensitization, even irritation or allergic reactions in consumers.

The color of lipsticks can be modulated by a degree of transparency. Lipsticks can thus range from "natural" near colorless or slight coloring to high coverage in their applied layer on lips. Titanium dioxides are sometimes used to increase coverage, but they also introduce a whitening effect on the resulting lip shade due to their white initial color. These particles also need special attention due to their mattifying effect on a formulation, which can counter an expected gloss or high shine expectation. Color is imparted by absorbing dye pigments such as D&C dyes. Additional optical effects can be introduced by means of interference pigments (based on silica, mica, borosilicates) reflecting selective color wavelengths. The size of these pigments plays an important role, since larger particles give a glitter effect but finer particles can bring a silky appearance to a lip product. Interference pigments (positive color component system) can often contrast with darker base colors of a lipstick. For example, fine golden interference pigments, bring a warm tone to a darker red/ochre lipstick. Typical colorant concentrations range from 4 to 20%.

c. Gloss ingredients

Lipsticks and lip-glosses are often intended to bring high gloss and shine when applied on lips. This is generally obtained by use of oils, esters, and silicones helping to form a homogeneous coating on lips and enhancing the light reflection by increasing the refractive index of the lipstick film. These ingredients also help the cohesion of a formulation, especially when using fillers and larger pigments that disrupt the cohesion of a lipstick during molding.

d. Oils

Many oils can be used in lipsticks, such as castor oil, mineral oils, and hydrogenated vegetable oils. Their viscosity ranges from liquid to near wax-like, and they play a role of dispersant for colorants as well as cohesion enhancer in lipsticks. Excessive amounts can lead to heavy feel, rancidity, or too much payoff when lipsticks are being applied by a consumer. Many oils need a co-solvent such as fatty alcohols to ensure their good dissolution in a formulation. Typical oil concentrations range from 6 to 10%.

e. Waxes

The most commonly used waxes in lipsticks are beeswax and Carnauba wax. Generally, waxes are used to increase the viscosity of a lipstick and balance the effects of oils and esters. Waxes are harder ingredients and they raise the melting point of a formulation. This control in the melting temperature of the lipstick also controls the payoff of a lipstick, which is the amount of product transferred from the lipstick to the lips of a consumer. Payoff needs to be adjusted based on the amount of colorants and the expected degree of coverage. Excessive use of waxes can lead to tackiness, graininess, and unpleasant application feel. Typical wax concentrations range from 8 to 18%.

f. Solvents

Alcohols and esters are generally used as solvents to disperse color pigments and waxes. Many esters are available for this: linear and branched alkyl esters, and from stearates (e.g., glyceryl-, iso-, hydroxyl-stearates) to palmitates, lanolin alcohols, caprylates, and others. Typical solvent concentrations range from 3 to 10%.

g. Silicones

These ingredients can range from liquids to wax-like consistency. They bring a lighter feel to the lipstick and decrease the greasy/heavy perception for consumers. Polar esters are often used as co-solvent with silicones. Typical concentrations range from 1 to 5%.

h. Polymers

Polymers are used to impart film-forming properties to lipsticks as well as to ensure the global film cohesion once applied onto lips. Another critical benefit of polymers is wear resistance. Usually, a large-scale polymer is used for film adhesion and flexibility to follow the movements of the lips while a finer-branched polymer serves to create the three-dimensional local network inside the film and traps colorant dyes, preventing their release on textiles or drinking containers (glass, ceramics). Polymers such as an acrylate/C_{12-22} alkylmethacrylate copolymers also provide good adhesion of the lipstick during application on lips. Finally, polymers can contribute to gloss in a lipstick by improving the quality of the film on lips and/or by increasing the refractive index of the lipstick [6].

Typical polymer concentrations range from 0.2 to 2%.

i. Additional ingredients

Sunscreens are often included in lipstick products to bring a protection against ultraviolet light. Sun-protection factors range typically from 8 to 15. These ingredients are generally oils, so higher amounts of waxes are used to counter their lowering of viscosity. A good dispersion of sunscreen filters can be obtained by alcohol co-solvents.

Moisturizing ingredients such as glycerol are sometimes used in lipsticks. Adding a moisturizer helps maintain the skin condition but also the fullness of lips and thus more attractiveness.

Antioxidants are sometimes used in lipsticks at lower concentrations (0.1–1%) and intended to remove ultraviolet-induced radicals inside the skin of lips.

Numerous fragrances can be used in lipsticks to give a fruity smell/taste to products or sometimes to mask heavier greasy ingredients of less appealing perception.

6.8.4 MASCARAS

The formulation of mascaras has been a very active field over the last 20 years as formulations are requested to improve very different aspects of eye lashes: color, physical characteristics such as curling and thickening, and daily wear resistance such as water and sweat resistance [7]. These effects can be almost instantly experienced and judged by the consumer, since mascara has a direct impact on visual perception. One must also keep in mind when formulating, that mascara formulations need to be adjusted to the applicator used in a final product, especially in terms of viscosity and application fluidity versus solvent evaporation.

Mascara formulations are found of two main types: water based and organic-solvent based. Both types can give smooth and homogenous applications on eye-lashes. Also, a very important aspect of mascaras is that formulations need to be matched with applicator brushes. This point is illustrated by the numerous patents existing on mascara applicator brushes [8–11].

a. Basic formulation

A general composition breakdown of mascaras is given in Table 26.1 as a base of discussion to follow.

Table 26.1 Typical mascara ingredients and ranges of commonly used concentrations

Ingredient	Concentration (% wt.)	Examples
Color	1–12%	iron oxide, mica pigments
Emulsifier	3–10%	myristoyl penta/hexapeptides
Emollients	25–50%	oils (jojoba, wheat, argan)
Texture modifiers	5–20%	hydroxycellulose, waxes
Preservative	0–1.5%	phenoxyethanol, propylparaben
Film formers	1–8%	silicones, dimethicone
Solvent	Q.S.	water, petroleum distillates

The primary purpose of a mascara is to give visual impression of long dark eyelashes to enhance the beauty of the eye area. Therefore, a first component will be the color pigments. For a best contrast of the visibility of eyelashes against the background skin and eye, black is the most common primary pigment and is given by black iron oxide particles. Titanium dioxide is often added to disperse black pigments and give a deeper black perception The main color can be modified as a mass-tone color by addition of light-absorption pigments such as browns, reds, and blue pigments (e.g., mica-based pigments). Two types of light-effect pigments can be used: light-absorbing (dye pigments) and light-reflecting/interfering (multicoated interference pigments). The second type is generally used in mascaras for its better perception due to selective color of light being reflected but also due to the lower toxicity of mica and its outer coating when in contact with eyelid skin and the humid mucosal membrane hosting lash roots.

Stronger mascara colors are also present on the market and represent a smaller fraction of consumer uses.

Emulsifiers are then added to create a stable dispersion of these pigments.

Thickeners such as hydroxyethylcellulose serve to thicken this suspension and can add volume to the mascara coating applied to the eyelash. They have a wide compatibility with most formulation bases, and while being commonly used, they also increase viscosity so that the system needs to be a little more fluidized (e.g., oils or emollients) for a smooth flow of mascara application.

Oils are commonly present to bring both better adhesion on the keratin of the lash keratin surface but also to fluidize the formulation to regularize flow and homogeneity during application. Oils also bring nourishment to the lash fiber by slightly penetrating into its cortex. Thickeners, such as waxes, have an opposite effect on the formulation by increasing viscosity but also induce a slight solidification of the mascara film during drying on eyelashes as the solvent evaporates. For this reason, it is generally recommended to move the applicator brush up and down in mascara tubes prior to use. The effect is to coat the locality, refluidize the formulation, and have a fresh layer of formulation on the brush when used. The same is recommended when using mascara consecutively.

b. Advanced ingredients

Specialty ingredients can be included to give a better texture or regularity when applied with a brush as well as additional benefits: adhesion promoters, formulation stabilizers, thickeners, polymers, color pigments, active ingredients, and fragrance. These ingredients are more and more frequently added to enhance the mascara film formation and stability on the eyelash and to bring new benefits to the final formula, such as water and wear resistance.

A detailed water-based mascara formulation is shown in Formula 26.6 below. This formulation has been shown to bring lash curling and water resistance but also a modest increase in lash thickness (volumizing effect).

Formula 26.6. Volume curling mascara with high water resistance

Phase	Ingredients	% (wt)
A	D.I. WATER	45.42
	Disodium EDTA (Versene Na2 Crystal)	0.1
	Triethanolamine (TEA 99%)	0.38
	Acrylic acid/VP Crosspolymer (Ultrathix p-100)	0.5
	Xantham gum (Keltrol T)	0.3
B	Water	10
	Polyninyl pyrrolidone (PVP-K30)	1
C	Iron oxide (Unipure black LC989)	12
D	Glyceyl stearate and Laureth-23 (CERASYNT 945)	3
	C_{18-36} acid triglyceride (Synchrowax HGLC)	5
	White beeswax	5
	Stearic acid	2
	Copernicia cerifera (Carnauba) wax SP63	3
	Euphorbia cerifera (Candelilla) wax	1
	PEG-20 stearate (Lipo PEG10-S)	2
	Tricontanyl PVP (Ganex WP-660)	0.5
E	Triethanolamine (TEA 99%)	1
F	Water	5
	Allantoin	0.1
	Vitamin E (Tocopheryl acetate)	0.2
	Acrylate/alkylmethacrylate copolymer (Allianz OPT)	1
G	Phenoxyethanol, octanediol (optiphen)	1.5
	Total:	100

Procedure

1. Pre-weigh water and disodium EDTA and mix until clear; add TEA and mix until clear. Sprinkle Ultrathix slowly until all in.
2. Transfer to homomixer and slowly add xantham gum.
3. Premix ingredients of phase B and add to phase A; begin heating to 75–80°C

4. Weigh ingredients of phase C and pulverize using blender for about five minutes. Then, add to previous mixture and continue homogenizing.
5. Separately, add ingredients of phase D and heat to 75–80°C while mixing.
6. Add phase D to phases ABC while homogenizing for about ten minutes.
7. Add TEA (phase E) and continue homogenizing for ten minutes. Begin cooling the mixture to 55°C.
8. Switch to sweep agitation. Add phases F and G and cool to 25–30°C.

Adhesion promoters such as silicones improve film compatibility of the mascara with the keratin of the eyelash cuticles. Adhesives help to prevent mascara flaking under daily stresses such as finger contact or bending or inter-eyelash friction. Stabilizers are used as homogenizers in the mascara. Thickeners such as hydroxyl celluloses provide richer coating applications on the lash and can thus bring volumizing properties to the finished product. Mechanical benefits such as anti-flaking or water resistance can be given to a formulation via polymers such as Allianz OPT or Ganex line. They provide two benefits to the mascara film applied on the eyelash: trapping of dyes and global film integrity. They give hold to the mascara dye particles by forming a three-dimensional network around them and throughout the film and thus prevent their release when lashes come in contact with waterous media such as tears. In addition, polymers give film integrity to the mascara while still adapting to the bending stress of eyelashes during daily activities. This prevents mascara breakage with risk of dye leakage or potential flaking of the film.

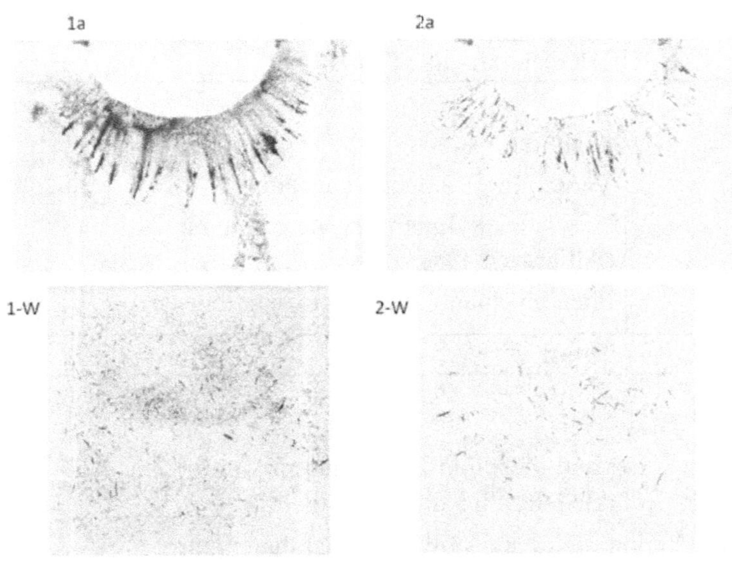

Figure 26.5. Effect of 1% acrylate/C_{12}–C_{22} alkyl methacrylate copolymer on water resistance: Test 1 (Top): Bending under wet conditions and Test 2 (Bottom):

particles released after 60 seconds of eyelash immersion in deionized water. (1) Mascara base without polymer; (2) mascara with 1% acrylate/C_{12}–C_{22} alkyl methacrylate copolymer. In all cases, mascara was applied on eyelashes and given 20 minutes drytime at air prior to tests.

Much work is devoted by finished product manufacturers to prescreen and test polymers and polymer mixtures for they glassy transition temperature, i.e., the temperature at which the material transitions from liquid to an amorphous glass-like state. A polymer mixture with a transition temperature near 68°F (20°C) would provide stability and luster to the applied mascara. The same polymers can also bring curling to a mascara (Figure 26.6)

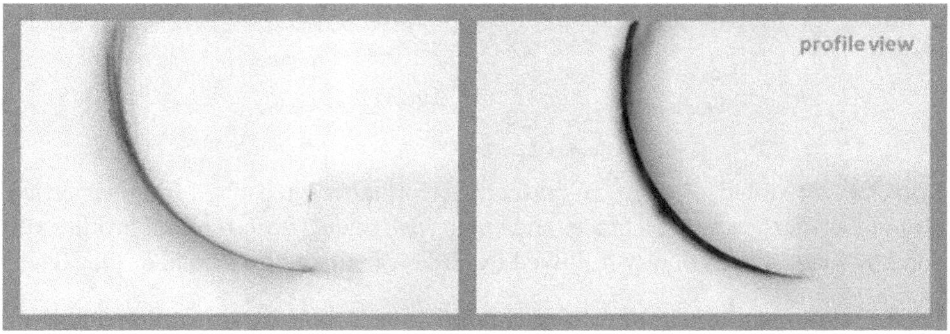

Figure 26.6. Side view of eyelashes before and after two-stroke application of formulation 1. Artificial eyelashes made of natural untreated Caucasian hair have been used here, mounted in a linear holder to control base hair alignment. The increase in curvature can be clearly seen on the right picture.

A multidimensional approach to polymer benefits in mascaras can serve the formulator to choose appropriate ingredients faster. A large number of commercial polymers have been evaluated in the mascara base at 1% active concentration (Formula 26.5). Four properties of mascaras have been evaluated as described above: volume, curling, water resistance, and shine. Results are graphed together on a spider chart to show best combinations of polymers providing multiple benefits to consumers. For each property, scales were normalized with the top performer in each category. For comparison, the six top-selling commercial mascaras were also tested. While most commercial products show very good performance in one property, only two of them showed two benefits at a high level. In comparison, 1% triacontanyl PVP showed high water resistance as well as curling and some degree of shine. In a 0.5% combination of triacontanyl PVP with 0.5% AOPT, all three properties were brought up to 80% of the highest performances.

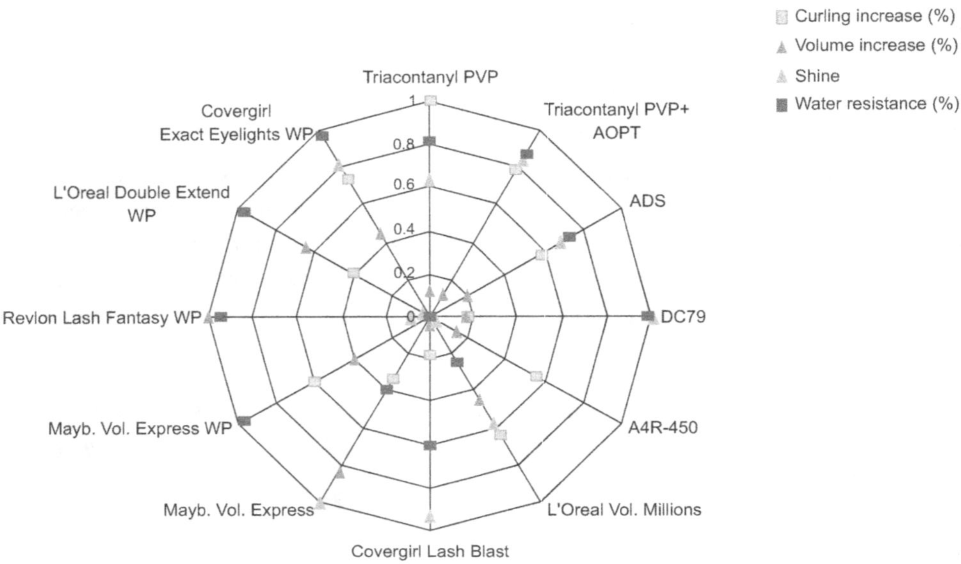

Figure 26.7. Global overview of mascara performances in each of four properties: volume, curling, water resistance, and shine (calculated from ten line profiles obtained by macrophotography followed by shine calculated by means of the Reich-Robbins formula)

Color pigments, such as micas, can bring highlights and color shades to the applied mascara. Finally, active ingredients can be incorporated inside mascaras or mascara pretreatments for various purposes such as reinforcing thin lashes or stimulating lash growth. Growth-stimulating actives are intended to penetrate into the lash follicle and act on the cell keratinization and differentiation.

6.8.5 SKINCARE ACTIVES IN FOUNDATIONS AND LIPSTICKS

The most common skin-active ingredients found in foundations and lipsticks are sunscreens. Numerous examples can be found where both types of products also claim sunscreen protection. Daily wear products now generally incorporate sunscreen filters against UVB and UVA. Very often, filters will be minerals such as titanium dioxide and zinc oxide, since organic filters tend to bind and react with oxide pigments. Another concern of organic filters is their absorption by pigments, which potentially leads to a decrease in SPF value. Mineral sunscreens have the advantage of dispersing well within the formulation and the application on skin while behaving neutral towards pigments. They are often used to achieve SPF values of 15–20 with concentrations of 10% w.

An additional skin care benefit brought to those products is moisturization. Commonly, glycerol is used in those cases but it also brings a slight drop in viscosity of the bulk formula as well as an oilier appearance when applied onto a person. This oily perception can be countered in foundations by either a slight increase in pigment fillers or by use of a polymer to give the product a finer visual texture instead of a local shine. However, it is less of a problem in lipsticks, since shine is an expected attribute. Lipsticks use a number of additional ingredients for moisturization and conditioning from oils (macademia, olive, castor seed, lavender, shea butter) to more complex natural ingredients (silk complex).

REFERENCES

1. Barel A. et al. Handbook of cosmetic science and technology., 3rd ed. CRC Press. 2009. Chapter 37.
2. Puccetti G. et al., Skin colorimetric parameters involved in skin perception. Skin Res. Technol. 2011, 1-6.
3. Korichi R., Video imaging in the measurement of makeup efficacy and performance. Cosmetics & Toiletries. 2002.
4. Burns R.S., Principles of Color Technology. 2000. Wiley-Interscience. Chapter 6.
5. Ackerman D. A natural history of the senses. 1991; Vintage Publishing.
6. Yadav S. et al., Luster measurements of lips treated with lipstick formulations. *Journal of the Society of Cosmetic Chemists*, Vol. 62, No. 3, 317-326.
7. Kwak T. et al. The character of eyelashes and the choice of mascara in Korean women. Skin Res. Technol. 2002.
8. Gueret J.-L. et al., US Patent #4887622. Brush for the application of mascaras to eyelashes. 1989.
9. Kingsford T., US Patent #5137038. Adjustable curve mascara brush. 1990.
10. Vasas M.M., US Patent #6237609B1. Curved longitudinal profile mascara brush. 2001.
11. Diaz L.F.H. US Patent # 6565276B1. Electrically driven handheld device for eyelash mascara application. 2003.

ABBREVIATIONS

AOPT, Acrylates/C12-22 Alkylmethacrylate copolymer; ADS, Vinyl Caprolactam/VP/Dimethylaminoethyl Methacrylate Copolymer; DC79, acrylates/acrylamide copolymer; A4R-450, PPG-17/IPDI/DMPA copolymer.

HAI R CARE

PART 6.9

FORMULATING WISDOM CATEGORY BY CATEGORY

Hair's original purpose was to provide body coverage and warmth—the first line of the body's defense against the environment. Hair has evolved to provide minimal protective function but becomes highly important in the areas of appearance and hygiene.

Composed of nonbiologically active protein, the hair has many unique and important properties—flexibility, extendability, insolubility (to normally experienced solvents), and adaptability (to changes in length, style, color, etc.). Hair grows at approximately 0.25–0.33 inches per month. Unlike living skin, hair cannot repair itself—whatever damage occurs remains until the hair is lost naturally by shedding, is cut, or breaks off.

The products developed for hair care serve multiple purposes—cleaning, conditioning, treating, coloring, etc. The following is a description of the categories involved in hair care.

PART 6.10

SHAMPOOS
INGREDIENTS, FORMULATION AND EFFICACY EVALUATION

Author
Carrie Shipley
Applications Scientist
Grain Processing Corporation

ABSTRACT

When formulating a successful shampoo, there are many components and interactions to take into consideration. This chapter will begin with Section I by introducing some of the basic ingredients used in the formulation of shampoos as well as what differentiates some of the types of shampoos on the market. The subsequent section will discuss the actual cleansing mechanism of shampoos and the effects that shampoos and surfactants have on the hair. Section III introduces a few of the factors used to evaluate a shampoo formulation as well as some of the key attributes that need to be taken into consideration when evaluating a shampoo's performance. The final section wraps up with a brief look into the future trends of the shampoo industry.

TABLE OF CONTENTS

INTRODUCTION

It would seem that modern day shampoos have come a long way from the first commercial shampoos that were introduced in the early 20th century, and in many respects, they have. Modern formulations have become more personalized, less harsh, and tend to follow certain consumer-driven trends. On the other hand, shampoos cannot stray far from their origination because design designates them to do one primary function: clean the hair and scalp.

When formulating a successful shampoo, there are many components and interactions to take into consideration. The surfactant system may seem to be the most important part of the formulation due to the primary functionality of a shampoo. It is very important to use a carefully chosen blend of surfactants that will deliver the appropriate detergency, lather, and wetability to a formula, but this should not delineate from the importance of the other ingredients in a shampoo formulation. Consumers have certain expectations from their shampoos. They expect a certain viscosity and rheology as well as other benefits such as good combability, shine, and manageability.

In the following sections, this chapter will outline some of the basic ingredients used to formulate different types of shampoos as well as examples of starting formulas. A detailed explanation of how these ingredients clean the hair and scalp as well as the effect that they can have on hair will be discussed. The final sections focus on evaluation components for shampoo formulas as well as for performance attributes and end with a brief look into the future of the shampoo industry.

SECTION I: TYPICAL SHAMPOO INGREDIENTS

6.10.1 SURFACTANTS

The surfactant component of a formula provides many basic functions to a shampoo. Not only do these ingredients provide the cleansing mechanism for the shampoo, but surfactants also provide the foaming, contribute to the formulation rheology, and also play a large part in the safety of the shampoo. Foaming properties have to be adequate, both in quantity and quality, for the consumer to consider a shampoo to be adequate. Foam does not equal quality to a formulator, but to a consumer, copious amounts of rich foam are a basic expectation for a good shampoo.

Shampoo formulations usually consist of primary as well as secondary surfactants. The primary surfactants are responsible for the main cleansing mechanism in the formula as well as the foaming and some of the viscosity control. Secondary surfactants are usually gentler than the primary surfactants but by themselves do not have the best foaming or cleansing properties. These surfactants are usually added to help boost the foaming and detergency as well as reduce irritation caused by many primary surfactants. Most primary surfactants in shampoos (not including baby shampoos or special formulations) are anionic or negatively charged molecules, while most secondary surfactants are nonionic (have no charge), amphoteric (can be positive or negative depending on pH), or cationic (positively charged).

Anionic Surfactants

Alkyl and alkyl either sulfates are the most commonly used primary surfactants in the majority of shampoos on the market. These surfactants are excellent cleansers and foamers. They are cost effective and can easily be thickened with sodium chloride, which makes them a popular choice for many shampoo formulations. Most mainstream formulations contain some combination of alkyl and/or alkyl ether sulfate with sodium lauryl sulfate (SLS), sodium laureth sulfate (SLES), ammonium lauryl sulfate (ALS), and ammonium laureth sulfate (ALES) being the most prevalent.

The lauryl and laureth sulfates are produced by a sulfation reaction using mostly C_{12} fatty alcohols. This chain length is chosen to maximize the foaming and wetting traits of the final surfactant. Various mixes of C_{12}–C_{14} chain lengths are commonly used but will vary depending on the manufacturer [1].

As stated above, SLS and ALS are excellent foamers and cleansers, but many of the 12 carbon chain-length fatty alcohols can cause irritation to the scalp and eyes and have some solubility issues. This is reduced by the reaction of the fatty alcohols with ethylene oxide (EO) prior to the sulfation process, producing SLES as well as ALES. The higher the degree of ethoxylation, the more soluble the compound as well as the higher the reduction of irritation is seen. SLES is usually reacted with an average of two moles of EO while ALES is commonly ethoxylated to an average three moles of EO.

The lauryl and laureth sulfates are sometimes used by themselves but are most commonly used in combination with each other. Lauryl sulfates by themselves produce a creamier foam with smaller bubbles while laureth sulfates produce better flash foam. When used in combination, they complement each other. When deciding between the sodium and ammonium salts, ALS/ALES produce a slightly higher amount of foam and can be easier to thicken, but care has to be taken when using these surfactants because they can release free ammonia at higher pH values.

Although most mainstream shampoos will have some sort of alkyl or alkyl ether sulfate combination as their primary surfactant base, alpha olefin sulfonates (AOS) rank second in use [2]. The alpha olefin sulfonates are usually 14 to16 carbons in length and are comparable to SLS and SLES in foaming capacity (in the presence of sebum). AOS is easily solubilized and contains very little color or odor. It is stable over a wide pH range including lower pH systems, which is a benefit over the alkyl and alkyl ether sulfates. In lower pH formulations, alkyl and alkyl ether sulfates can be hydrolyzed. AOS is usually not used in premium shampoos because it has been reported to leave a harsher feel than the lauryl or lauryl sulfates and is also harder to thicken. Due to AOS surfactants containing a sulfonate group instead of a sulfate group, these surfactants can be formulated into sulfate-free formulas.

Other Anionic Surfactants

Sulfosuccinates. Sulfosuccinates contain both a carboxylate and a sulfonate group and are often used in combination with alkyl and alkyl ether sulfates in mild shampoo formulations or as part of a surfactant combination in baby shampoo formulas. The addition of a sulfosuccinate surfactant helps reduce eye and skin irritation, improves the lather, and contributes some conditioning benefits.

N-Acyl Methyltaurates. N-acyl methyltaurates (AMT) are the fatty amides of methyltaurines. They are noted for their low irritancy and are claimed to protect hair against cuticle damage. This class of surfactants finds limited usage in shampoos because of poor solubility and foaming performance, especially in hard water [3].

Sarcosinates. N-acyl sarcosinates are produced by reacting a fatty acyl chloride with N-methylglycine. These secondary surfactants do not lather well and tend to form precipitates in hard water, but are extremely mild. They can be used in combination with other anionic surfactants to reduce eye and skin irritation as well as provide some conditioning properties. The two most common forms of this surfactant that are used in shampoos is cocoyl sarcosinate and sodium lauryl sarcosinate [4].

Isethionates. Acyl Isethionates are condensation products of fatty acid chlorides and the sodium salt of 2-hydroxyethanesulfonic acid. They are very mild to the scalp and hair and produce a creamy, soap-like lather in both soft and hard water. They hydrolyze easily at low and high pHs. They have limited solubility at room temperature and so are not used in clear formulations [3].

N-acyl polypeptide condensates (protein derivatives). This class of surfactants is produced by the condensation of fatty acid chlorides and low-molecular-weight protein hydrolysates. Most often the cation is either potassium or triethanolamine, and the acyl group is a cocoyl moiety [3]. These surfactants have poor flash-foaming properties but produce a creamy, tight lather. They are stable in hard water, very mild to the eyes and skin, and have some conditioning attributes, but can be susceptible to bacteria [5].

Nonionic Surfactants

Although the detergency of nonionic surfactants is equal to, and in many instances superior to, that of anionic surfactants, nonionics are generally not used as primary surfactants in shampoos. This is due to inferior foaming characteristics, which result from their large surface area per molecule and the lack of charge on the surface films in nonionic foams [1]. However, nonionics are used extensively in a secondary capacity as foam modifiers, viscosity builders, emulsifiers, solubilizing aids, and in some case, conditioning agents.

Alkanolamides

One of the most common classes of nonionic surfactants is the fatty alkanolamides. They are produced by the condensation of a mixture of a primary or secondary alkanolamine with a fatty acid or derivative. The ratio of the amine to fatty acid yields differing products. The 1:1 condensates, referred to as "superamides," are much more prevalent in shampoo formulations. Products derived from different fatty derivatives and different condensation ratios carry the same name, and wide variations in the chemical composition and performance of Alkanolamides from different manufacturers is not unexpected [3].

Alkanolamides are used for foam stabilization as well as viscosity enhancement, but care has to be used when choosing the alkanolamide to formulate with. Many formulators shy away from formulating with cocamide DEA or diethanolamine due to the potential for free amine production, which can form carcinogenic N-nitosamines. Many formulators will use Cocamide MEA (monoethanolamine), which is the monomer form. The foam stability is comparable to that of the DEA form, but the MEA form will build slightly higher viscosity.

Amine Oxides

Another widely used class of nonionic surfactant, the amine oxides are prepared by the oxidation of tertiary amines with hydrogen peroxide. The N-O bond is highly polarized, and at below-neutral pHs, amine oxides become protonated, which allows them to take on cationic characteristics such as conditioning and anti-static benefits. At pH 7 and above, the molecule is nonionic. The performance of an amine oxide can be compared to that of an alkanolamide. Amine oxides are best known for their ability to enhance foam characteristics and stabilize lather as secondary surfactants [3].

Alkyl Polyglucosides

One of the newer nonionic classes of nonionic surfactants are the alkyl polyglucosides. These can be considered hybrids combining properties from nonionic and anionic surfactants. They are prepared by reacting corn starch glucose with a fatty alcohol. The result is group of surfactants that are good foamers, have good detergency and wetting properties, and are toxicologically safe and biodegradable [1]. They are mostly used as secondary surfactants to help reduce irritation from the primary surfactant.

Polyethoxylated Surfactants

These surfactants represent the largest group of nonionics and include fatty alcohols, the ethoxylated derivatives of alkylphenols, fatty esters, and diglycerides. They have poor foaming power but are excellent cleansers, which makes them unusable in many shampoos as a primary surfactant. When used as secondary surfactants, both polysorbate-20 and PEG-80 sorbitan laurate can greatly reduce eye irritation caused by anionic surfactants and will not affect the foaming attributes

[1]. It is because of these reasons that these nonionic surfactants are usually formulated into baby shampoos.

Amphoterics

Amphoterics can be divided into two groups based on their pH response. The first group contains the carboxylated imidzoles and N-alkyl betaines. This group is zwitterionic at pHs at and above their isoelectric points and cationic at lower pHs. The second group contains the sulfobetaines and phosphobetaines, which are zwitterionic as the anionic portion is dissociated at all pHs [1]. The amphoterics have a very low irritation potential and are almost completely nonstinging to the eyes. These surfactants are compatible with a wide range of other surfactants and can be formulated into many different types of shampoos including baby shampoos. For instance, they are often found in conditioning shampoos due to their compatibility with quaternary compounds.

It should be noted that true amphoterics actually contain dual functional groups in the same molecule that allows them to exist in nonionic, cationic, as well as anionic states depending on pH. Betaines exist only in their nonionic and cationic states, depending on pH [1]. Betaines function as excellent foam boosters and viscosity enhancers when utilized as secondary surfactants, having good water solubility over a wide pH range [3]. Cocamidopropyl betaine is the most widely used example of this type of amphoteric surfactant and is often used in amide-free formulas as well as baby shampoos.

Cationic Surfactants

For several reasons, the use of cationic (positively charged) surfactants in shampoo formulations is more limited than that of other surfactant classes. They are generally not as effective detergents due to their ability to strongly bind to the hair's negatively charged surface. Their foaming properties are inferior to those of anionics. Furthermore, because they are not efficiently removed during rinsing, the hair is left more hydrophobic with the cationic's hydrophobic tail extending from the surface. This results in increased attraction of oily soils to the hair. Therefore, their use (at low levels) has been limited to their hair conditioning, lubricating, and antistatic benefits [3].

6.10.2 RHEOLOGY AND VISCOSITY MODIFIERS

Surfactants are fundamental to the formulation of a shampoo, but the rest of the ingredients should not be overlooked. Many of these ingredients play an important role in how a shampoo is viewed by the consumer. A surfactant blend diluted in water cleans just fine, but the average person won't be convinced of this. The consumer is conditioned to look for certain attributes in a shampoo, and much of the initial perception of a shampoo's cleaning ability is dependent upon the rheology and viscosity of the formula.

Shampoo rheology and viscosity are difficult to discuss independently. Rheology and viscosity are not interchangeable terms, but rheology, or the flow properties of a product, cannot be determined without taking into consideration viscosity or thickness, of non-Newtonian fluids such as shampoos. Viscosity modifiers have their own rheology, which must be taken into consideration when used to thicken because they are going to lend some of these rheological characteristics to the final formula. Some of the common viscosity modifiers are going to be discussed as well as the rheology they contribute to the final shampoo formula.

Salts

The most common way to add viscosity to a surfactant system is by adding a salt. While salt is not necessarily a viscosifier in the same means as the other reagents that will be discussed, salts are one of the most common substances often used in conjunction with other agents (salt-responsive thickeners), to control viscosity and modify rheology in anionic and nonionic surfactant systems. Sodium chloride is a commonly used monovalent salt in this process, but multivalent salts can be used also and are more effective since they contribute more ionic strength to the solution. Divalent salts such as calcium and magnesium chloride are not used as often because they tend to precipitate out and raise the cloud point of a shampoo formula. Ammonium chloride is another commonly used multivalent salt and is very effective, but pH and concentration have to be taken into consideration, especially if using an ammonium-based surfactant. Free ammonia can be given off if formulated above a neutral pH.

Salts themselves do not provide the thickening mechanism but in conjunction with surfactants, they promote a thickening of the surfactant system. Surfactants contain molecules with hydrophilic as well as hydrophobic portions. When specific surfactant concentrations are introduced to water, micellular structures are formed. These structures have hydrophilic or polar heads that orient themselves together in the water, while the hydrophobic tail regions sequester themselves in the center of the structure away from the water. These micelles are constantly moving and rearranging themselves. When salt is added to an anionic, nonionic, or some anionic-amphoteric surfactant systems, the charge density of the solution is lowered; this allows the micelles to pack more closely together, forming micellular agglomerates. These large agglomerates are what increase the viscosity of the shampoo. This mechanism does not work exactly the same in every formula. The salt-thickening response depends on the type and concentration of surfactants as well as the type of electrolyte used. Solution temperature and initial charge density of the formula also has to be considered [9]. Most surfactants already contain a small amount of free organic salts, so there is already some electrolyte present in the system, which can affect the amount of salt needed.

Salt addition is not always a simple way to thicken a surfactant system. Too much salt can create a phenomenon called "salting out." A small amount of electrolyte (usually between 0.1 and 3%) is needed to thicken most systems. Salting out happens when the maximum electrolyte balance has been reached and the amount of free electrolyte starts to interfere with the micelle structure. The charge density is then lowered and the micelles begin to repel each other, which dramatically decreases viscosity. The proper amount of electrolyte can be determined by plotting a salt curve using increments of 0.1% electrolyte and then taking a viscosity measurement [10]. It is important to stay on the upside of the curve in order to achieve maximum results. The ideal amount of salt will provide a Newtonian rheology to a shampoo formula. Too much salt can also create an undesirable rheology, which can be stringy and pituitous.

Alkanolamides

Foam-stabilizing agents such as alkanolamides (i.e., cocamide DEA, MEA) are discussed earlier in this chapter under the surfactant section. These agents are often added to shampoo formulas not only to create longer-lasting foam and a tighter structure, but also to build viscosity and modify the rheology of a shampoo formulation. These are salt-responsive thickeners. They will add a pseudoplastic rheology and provide thickening by interacting with the surfactant micelle [11]. This interaction shifts the salt curve, allowing less salt to be used to achieve maximum viscosity.

Acrylic Acid Polymers

Another group of commonly used viscosity builders and rheology modifiers used in shampoos are the acrylic acid polymers. This group includes, but is not limited to, carbomers, and acrylate crosspolymers and copolymers. Acrylic acid polymers are high-molecular-weight synthetic polymers that have the ability to swell in aqueous solutions. This swelling of the high-molecular-weight polymer is what provides the thickening mechanism. They cannot swell, however, without being neutralized by a base that converts them to their salt form. This can be done by the addition of NaOH, NH_4OH, or KOH. Acrylic acid polymers are very efficient thickeners that impart a highly pseudoplastic rheology. These polymers are normally compatible with most surfactants including cationics, but most have some amount of electrolyte and pH sensitivity [11].

Gums

Gums are frequently used to modify viscosity and rheology in shampoos. There are many gums available, but only a few that are commonly used in shampoo formulations. One of the most common, nonmodified gums used is Xanthan. Xanthan is enzymatically produced from the bacteria Xanthomonas campestis and is considered a natural thickener/rheology modifier. It is compatible with anionic and nonionic surfactants and also with most mono- and divalent salts. When used in very small amounts (0.1–0.5%), it provides sufficient thickening and a pseudoplastic flow [11]. When used in excess, Xanthan can have a very negative impact on rheology. The solution can turn to a soft gel upon standing and the flow becomes very elastic.

Gums can be modified to create certain characteristics, enhance solubility, or create a specific rheology. Cationic and hydroxypropyl guar (HP guar) are examples of modified guar gum. Cationic guar is substituted with a quaternary ammonia compound. The cationic portion of the molecule is substantive, so it creates a conditioning feel while the guar portion provides the thickening and rheological attributes. The HP guar is hydroxypropylated, which provides better pH and electrolyte stability.

Corn Starches

Using corn starch is another way to thicken a shampoo while controlling the rheology. Unfortunately, unmodified corn starch is rarely used as a viscosity control agent in personal care products due to its unmodified characteristics. Unmodified dent corn will retrograde and form opaque gels, and it also imparts a high viscosity during processing, which makes it hard to work with. Waxy corn, which is also a base commonly used to make corn starch, won't retrograde to the same extent as a dent corn–based starch due to its high amylopectin content, but it has a very stringy, uneven flow that is not favored for a shampoo. Most corn starch that is used for rheology modification is chemically and or physically modified. These modifications (primarily hydroxypropylation) help create starches with increased clarity, less retrogradation, lower gelatinization temperatures, greater pH toleration, and the ability to help with foam stability due to increased film-forming capabilities. The addition of modified starch to a shampoo formula can add a short, thixotropic rheology to a shampoo and will enhance spreadability.

Corn starches are made up of small granules that swell when hydrated. This mechanism is what causes an increase in viscosity. When added into a solution containing a high amount of surfactant such as a shampoo, the surfactant can interfere with the swelling of the granules by grabbing up the available water, causing a decrease in normal viscosity development as well as an upward shift in the gelatinization temperature. The situation is dependent on the starch base as well as the type of surfactant used. This may be linked to the amount of amylose contained in the starch granule [12]. Waxy maize starches with very little if any amylose tend to see less of this phenomenon, whereas dent-based starches which contain roughly 24% amylose will see this decrease in viscosity. For the shampoo formulator using corn starch as a viscosity/rheology modifier, it is important to know this when formulating. As a rule of thumb, waxy-based corn starches will contribute higher viscosity with less usage but can have a slightly longer texture, dent-based corn starches require a higher usage but will contribute a shorter, smoother texture. Corn starches can also be used to thicken most cationic-based surfactants where some of the other viscosity modifiers fail.

Cellulose Derivatives

Cellulose derivatives are often used for viscosity control and rheology modification, but much like corn starch, are used in their modified form. Cellulose derivatives can be modified to be more or less hydrophilic as well as pH and electrolyte tolerant. Some of the most frequently used modified cellulosics are methylcellulose, hydroxypropyl methylcellulose, and hydroxyethylcellulose. They provide a pseudoplastic rheology and are typically used at 0.5–1.5% [11].

Modified Polyethylene Glycols

Modified polyethylene glycols (PEG) are nonionic thickeners that provide different rheologies depending on the R-group that is attached to the basic chemical structure. The R-groups can consist of either a fatty alcohol, a glyceryl ester, or a propylene glycol. Of these polymers, the most commonly used PEGs for shampoos are the stearic acid esters of polyethylene glycol, typically PEG-150 distearate. The number associated with the PEG denotes the number of PEG moles in the polymer. PEG-150 distearate is a high-molecular-weight polymer that is compatible with most surfactants as well as pH, and is temperature stable, which imparts a shear-thinning rheology to a shampoo formulation [11].

Others

Some of the other viscosity modifiers used in shampoos are clays such as bentonite, hectorite, and magnesium aluminum silicate. They impart a thixotropic rheology to a formula by swelling to produce viscosity. This group of thickeners can also be used to stabilize colloidal or pearl systems in shampoos as well as for stability in anti-dandruff shampoos.

6.10.3 OTHER SHAMPOO INGREDIENTS

Opacifiers and Pearlizing Agents

Opacity or pearlescence can be imparted to a shampoo by several different types of raw materials. Ethylene glycol stearate, glyceryl stearate, and cetyl or stearyl alcohols are frequently used with alkyl sulfates. These materials are incorporated into the surfactant solution at temperatures above their melting points and then crystallize upon cooling, producing a pearlescent appearance. The opacifying effect is dependent on the crystal size, distribution, and reflectance [3].

Antioxidants/Sequestrants/UV absorbers

Traditionally, antioxidants are included in shampoo formulations to avoid oxidation of unsaturated components such as vegetable oils and oleic acid derivatives. Typical antioxidants used are BHT, BHA, and tocopherol [3]. In some newer formulations, antioxidants have taken on a more modern role and have been marketed as helping to provide healthier hair by fighting free radicals. The antioxidants used in these shampoos are more often of the "superfruit" type.

Sequestering agents are included in shampoos to prevent the formation of insoluble metal ions, which can be formed in the presence of hard water. These ions can create a film on the hair, making it appear dull. The sequestering agent binds with the metals ions to form soluble complexes. Typically, EDTA and its salts, citric acid, or polyphosphates are used.

UV absorbers are not used in shampoo to the same degree and traditional sense as they once were. UV absorbers such as benzophenone are still used to protect formulations in clear packages against color fading or discoloration upon prolonged light exposure, but most shampoos manufactured today are contained in opaque packaging. When discussing UV absorbers in the present sense, most shampoo manufacturers market them as a protectant for the fading of hair color from light exposure. In order for a UV absorber to work in this way, it has to be water soluble as well as substantive to the hair. There are newer compounds available that combine quaternary ammonium compounds with UV filters to create this type of protection (multifunctional ingredients). One such ingredient is cinnamidopropyltrimonium chloride, which can be found on the ingredient statement of some shampoos and conditioners claiming color protection [6].

6.10.4 FRAGRANCE

Fragrance has become an increasingly important aspect of a shampoo formulation. The ability of a fragrance to influence consumers' perception of a shampoo should not be underestimated. The fragrance also serves the purpose of covering any base odor in the formula, particularly as the product ages. The level of fragrance incorporated into a shampoo formula above that necessary to cover base odor depends primarily on the intended shampoo market. The fragrance must be compatible with the shampoo formula, it should not adversely affect viscosity or stability, nor should it induce irritation. Factors affecting fragrance selection include evaluations of the residual fragrance left on the hair following shampooing in addition to assessments of the fragrance in the package and during use [3].

6.10.5 PRESERVATIVES

Preservatives are essential components of a shampoo formulation to protect against microbial growth. Among the potential sources of microbial contamination are water supplies, improperly cleaned manufacturing equipment, and raw materials [3].

There are generally three types of commonly used preservatives: parabens, formaldehyde donors, and MIT (methylisothiazolinone) systems. All have been under public fire for one reason or another, but all usage is highly regulated by each country's government.

Parabens include the esters such as methyl, ethyl, and propylparaben. These are very active against fungi and are weaker against gram-negative bacteria. They are also only active in the water phase of a formulation and can be inactivated, either partially or fully, by strong hydrogen bonders such as polysorbates, cellulose derivatives, and proteins [7].

Formaldehyde was once a common preservative in cosmetic and personal care formulations, but is rarely used in its raw form due to its carcinogenic link. It is banned in the EU as well as in Japan. The formaldehyde donors (DMDM hydantoin, quaternium 15, imidazolidinyl urea, diazolidinyl urea) tend to give off a small amount of free formaldehyde, but it is in a much lower quantity and since they are effective in such small percentages, these preservatives are used in place of formaldehyde. The formaldehyde donors all have their different strengths and weaknesses, but most perform the strongest against bacteria and the weakest against fungi. Formaldehyde-releasing preservatives should not be used with protein derivatives as they are inactivated during condensation with the free amino groups.

MIT can be used alone or in combination with other isothiazolinones such as chloromethyl isothiazolinone. These are broad-spectrum biocides that perform well against both bacteria and fungi [7].

Other Additives

Many modern shampoos have additives that take them beyond the basic cleansing shampoo and suggest additional cosmetic benefits. Some of these additives include proteins such as hydrolyzed wheat protein, hydrolyzed silk or collagen, vitamins such as panthenol and biotin, moisturizers and humectants, oils and botanicals. All have been marketed as an added benefit to the hair and scalp. These are normally added at such small percentages that there is some question of their actual benefits.

6.10.6 TYPES OF SHAMPOOS

Basic Cleansing

The basic cleansing or clarifying shampoo formula is formulated to remove substantive residues from styling products as well as provide a deeper cleaning than some of the other formulas. They are usually formulated with higher levels of anionic surfactants to boost the cleaning potential. The following is a typical basic formula for a cleansing shampoo:

Cleansing Shampoo

Ingredient	% wt/wt
Sodium laureth sulfate	25.0
Cocamidopropyl betaine	7.0
Cocamide MEA	2.0
Fragrance	0.7
Preservative	0.5
Citric acid	q.s. pH 5.5–6.5
Sodium chloride	q.s. viscosity
Water	q.s. to 100

Mild/Baby

Baby shampoos and other mild formulas (children's shampoos) are formulated for gentleness, especially to the eyes. To achieve this, these products are formulated with higher levels of nonionic and amphoteric surfactants, which are less irritating than the alkyl and alkyl ether sulfates. As mentioned before, the presence of ethylene oxide reduces the irritation of the anionic surfactants, so Polysorbate 20 and PEG-80 (20 and 80 moles of ethylene oxide respectively) are often used as anti-irritants in baby shampoos.

Baby Shampoo

Ingredient	% wt/wt
PEG-80 sorbitan laurate	12.0
Sodium trideceth sulfate	5.0
Sodium lauroamphoacetate	5.0
PEG-120 methyl glucose dioleate	2.0
Cocamidopropyl hydroxysultaine	1.0
Fragrance	0.7
Preservative	0.5
Water	q.s. to 100

Source: Reference [3]

Conditioning/Two-in-One

Most shampoos on the market today have some type of conditioning agent in them even if they are not labeled as an actual two-in-one shampoo. This helps to improve the wet combability, and adds softness and shine to the hair. These formulas are more complex than a typical basic or cleansing shampoo since most of the conditioning agents are not soluble in water, and an emulsion has to be made (usually oil in water), which will require the addition of some type of emulsifying agent.

Silicones such as dimethicone, dimethiconol, amodimethicone, and dimethicone copolyol are frequently used in these types of formulas. Silicones provide light conditioning by forming a thin film on the surface of the hair. This type of conditioning is less than that seen by a separate conditioner, but is sufficient to improve aesthetics over that of a shampoo without a conditioner.

A number of non-silicone conditioning agents have been used in shampoos, either alone or as secondary conditioners in two-in-one formulations. Because of their compatibility with anionic surfactants, cationic polymers such as polyquaternium-10 and polyquaternium-7 are sometimes used in these types of formulas. Normally, these two cationic polymers can be very substantive to the hair and can form deposits, but due to complexes that are formed with the cationic polymer and anionic surfactant, this deposition is greatly reduced [1].

Below is an example of a two-in-one formula from U.S. Patent 6,007,802 [13] containing polyquaternium-10 and an anionic surfactant as well as a dimethicone.

Conditioning (Two-in-One) Shampoo

Ingredient	% wt/wt
Ammonium laureth sulfate (3 EO)	14.00
Cocamidopropyl betaine	2.70

Ingredient	% wt/wt
Polyquaternium-10	0.15
B8/C10 diester of adipic acid	0.30
Cocamide MEA	0.80
Cetyl alcohol	0.42
Stearyl alcohol	0.18
Carbapol 981	0.50
Dimethicone	1.00
Fragrance	0.37
DMDM hydantoin	0.37
Color solution (ppm)	64
Water	q.s. to 100

Source: Reference [2]

Anti-Dandruff

In the United States shampoos and non-shampoos containing an anti-dandruff agent are considered drugs. Similar controls over these preparations exist in other legislative areas. Active anti-dandruff ingredients that can be used in the United States, as well as claims that can be made, are governed by the FDA under 21CFR358 subpart H. There are only a few active ingredients approved for use in the U.S. See Table 29.1 for the list of ingredients as well as the approved percentages.

Table 29.1. Anti-Dandruff Ingredients

Active Ingredient	Allowable Usage (%)
Coal tar	0.5–5.0
Salicylic acid	1.8–3.0
Sulfur	2.0–5.0
Selenium sulfide	1.0
Zinc pyrithione	0.3–2.0
Ketoconozole	1.0
Climbazole	1.0–2.0

Source: 21CFR358.D.2013

Most anti-dandruff agents are water-insoluble so that when the hair is rinsed after shampooing, the insoluble particulates remain on the hair and scalp for further treatment. This insolubility makes the actives harder to formulate with. Anti-dandruff agents can be difficult to suspend due to high specific densities, but much work has been done to improve formulations so that many now contain milder surfactants and conditioning agents.

The Sulfate/Amide-Free Shampoo

Trends come and go in the personal care world, but shampoo manufacturers must succumb to the consumer. Sulfate- and sometimes amide-free shampoos have become more mainstream in the last few years. Once only seen in specialty salons, they are now seen on the common store shelves. As consumers begin to pay more attention to ingredients in the products they use, certain ingredients come under scrutiny; surfactants containing sulfates are one of them. Sulfate-free shampoos are not always easy to formulate because the surfactants can be harder to thicken and may not foam as well as other conventional surfactants. ALS/ALES and SLS/SLES are used because of their excellent foaming and cleansing properties as well as their low cost. They are easy to thicken with electrolytes or other conventional thickeners and are readily available. Surfactant companies are constantly coming out with new surfactants to meet the needs of the formulator. The following is an example of a sulfate- and amide-free shampoo formula.

Amide- and Sulfate-Free Shampoo

Ingredient	% wt/wt
A. Water	31.72
Disodium laureth sufocuccinate (40%)	27.68
Cocamidopropyl betaine	17.89
Ammonium cocoyl isethionate (30%)	13.92
Lauramine oxide	4.83
PEG-30 glyceryl cocoate	1.00
Polyquaternium-7	0.60
B. PEG-120 methyl glucose dioleate	1.91
C. Preservative	0.05
D. Citric acid (adjust final pH 6.0–6.5)	0.40

Source: Reference [13]

Shampoos with Cosmetic Benefits

Most mainstream shampoos sold on the market today have some sort of cosmetic benefit tied to them. Cosmetic benefits can range from the simple addition of a humectant for moisturization to the claim of added volume, increased shine, strengthening, or revitalizing. These shampoos have become very popular as the consumer has grown to expect more from a shampoo than just basic cleansing. Below is an example of a volumizing shampoo.

Volumizing Shampoo

Ingredient	**% wt/wt**
A. Water	24.50
B. Polyquaternium-4	0.25
C. Sodium chloride	2.50
D. Water	26.27
E. Sodium laureth sulfate (28% active)	42.90
F. Cocamidopropyl betaine (30% active)	3.34
G. DMDM hydantoin	0.24
H. Citric acid	q.s. to pH 6.0–6.5

Source: Reference [13]

SECTION II: HAIR-CLEANSING MECHANISM

This chapter has discussed the basic ingredients that are involved in the formulation of a shampoo as well as the different types of shampoos that are commonly formulated. This next section is an excerpt from chapter 29 of *Harry's Cosmeticology 8th Edition* that does an excellent job explaining how shampoos carry out the cleansing mechanism as well as their effects on hair.

The surfactants play the leading role in cleansing mechanism, so an understanding of how surfactants carry out their hair-cleansing function is necessary in order to assess the relative cleaning efficiencies of different surfactants and surfactant combinations. It is also important for determining how best to balance, in a formulation, the often-conflicting aims of optimum cleaning, foam, viscosity, actives deposition, mildness, and so forth.

The epicutical of hair is substituted and coated with material responsible in large part for the observed hydrophobicity of untreated hair surfaces. Because of their protein composition, however, these surfaces can also contain charged hydrophilic sites. For virgin hair, the observed isoelectric point is near 3.67, which ensures that the hydrophilic sites on this hair will carry a negative charge at the ordinary pH level of shampoos. The combination of negative charge and the hydrophobicity affects not only the type of soils and actives that bind to the hair but also the ease with which different soils are removed from the fiber surface.

Most consumer-bought shampoos are not going to be used on virgin hair. Most modern hair succumbs to numerous cycles of chemical treatment as well as exposure to sunlight. This will affect the cleaning mechanism of a shampoo due to the fact that the distribution of negatively charged sites on untreated hair is uneven, increasing from root to tip. This is a result of exposure to sunlight, which oxidizes cystine in the hair to cystine S-sulfonate and cysteic acid. In addition to oxidation by sunlight, hair can also be chemically oxidized as a result of perming, bleaching, or permanent dyeing. These treatments, all of which include oxidative steps, convert cystine to cysteic acid. The degree of resultant negative charge is generally greater than that from sunlight oxidation. In many cases after sufficient treatment, the entire hair surface can be converted from a hydrophobic to a hydrophilic character. This, of course, also affects deposition and removal of materials on the hair surface.

6.10.7 CLEANING OF SOLID PARTICULATES

For studies of hair-surface cleaning, it is convenient to divide possible soils into two types: solid particulates and oily or liquid deposits. Particulate soils can come from the environment or from hair care products. Examples of the latter include many anti-dandruff agents, while the former include carbon particles in the form of soot, clays, or rubber abraded from automobile tires.

In general, solids soils adhere to the hair surface through ionic or van der Waals forces. The ease of removing these soils from a surface in water depends on the relative affinities for each other of the water, soil, and substrate. A hydrophobic particle, for example, would be much easier to remove from a hydrophilic substrate than from a hydrophobic surface. This can be seen in the equation for the work of adhesion, Wa, which is defined as the free-energy change per unit area involved in removing a solid particle from a surface to which it is adhered:

$$Wa = \gamma PW + \gamma HW - \gamma PH$$

In the above equation, γ is the interfacial tension between any two surfaces, P represents the particle, H represents the hair surface, while W represents water. For hydrophobic particles, γHW would be larger and γPH would be smaller for hydrophobic surfaces than for hydrophilic substrates. The resultant larger work of adhesion indicates again that hydrophobic particles are more difficult to remove from hydrophobic than from hydrophilic surfaces.

Anionic and nonionic detergents can effect removal of particles from hair surfaces by adsorbing to these substrates with their hydrophobic portions in contact with surface and their hydrophilic heads oriented toward the water. This reduces γHW and, therefore, Wa. Similarly, binding of surfactant to a hydrophobic soil reduces γPW, effecting an additional decrease in the work of adhesion.

A more effective cleaning mechanism than the preceding results when anionic surfactants adsorb to solid particles and the surfaces to which they are adhered. Such adsorption effectively deposits negative charge on both soil and substrate, facilitating soil removal as a result of mutual charge repulsion. Since nonionics cannot impart a charge potential on surfaces, they are not in general as effective as anionic surfactants in cleaning soils.

6.10.8 CLEANING OF OILY SOIL

The second major class of soils found on hair is hydrophobic, or oily, soil that is liquid, at least at cleaning temperatures. Examples include sebum from the scalp, which is mostly liquid at body temperature; silicones, oils and waxes from hair care products; and lipids from skin cells. There are a number of possible detergency mechanisms for these types of soils, including rollback, emulsification, solubilization, and mesophase formation. These are discussed in the following sections.

Rollback Mechanism

The expression for work of adhesion in the previous section applies to oily soils as well as particulates. As with particulates, the more hydrophobic the liquid soil, the more difficult it is to remove from a hydrophobic substrate. Also as with particulates, detergents can effect soil removal of oils by adsorbing to the hair surface. In this case, the increased affinity of the surface for water permits the water to displace the oil droplet and simply roll it up. This process is termed the rollback mechanism. This mechanism is described quantitatively by Young's equation, which for aqueous systems is written as:

$$\gamma HW = \gamma HO + \gamma OW \cos \theta$$

where γ is the interfacial tension between two phases, H represents hair, *O* represents the oil phase, and W represents water. θ in the above equation is the contact angle between the soil and the hair surface; the lower this angle, the greater is the contact between the two phases.

It is implicit in Young's equation that adsorption of a surfactant to the hair surface, which lowers γHW, will increase the contact angle of the oil droplet. For sufficiently large increases in γHW, θ will increase to 180°, and the oil droplet will spontaneously separate from the hair surface. In practice, application of mechanical work during shampooing—for example, flexing and rubbing of hair—will help to completely remove those soils. Increased temperature also aids in soil removal, facilitating droplet roll-up by reducing soil viscosity and also by increasing rates of surfactant adsorption. These temperature effects are particularly important in view of the short cleaning times involved in the shampooing process.

Solubilization of Soils

The rollback process is the most important soil-removal mechanism for products that are highly diluted during cleaning, so that surfactants are present primarily in the form of monomers.

If surfactant concentration is sufficiently high during use, then soil removal can also proceed via solubilization. This is accomplished by surfactant aggregates called micelles, which form above a certain concentration termed the critical micelle concentration, or CMC. The surfactants in micelles are arranged so that the surfactant heads form a hydrophilic surface in contact with the water, while the tails are lined up in the micelle interior, forming a hydrophobic core.

Micelles solubilize soils by incorporation into the micellular structure. More polar soils are incorporated near the hydrophilic heads, while hydrophobic soils end up deep in the micelle interior. Kinetic investigations on fatty acid solubilization indicate that solubilization begins by diffusion of micelles to the soil surface, followed by surfactant adsorption onto the soil and incorporation of soil into the surfactant aggregate. The process ends by desorption of the soil containing micelle and diffusion away from the surface. The latter two steps were found to control the rate of the solubilization process. The critical micelle concentration for most anionic shampoo is about 5×10^{-3} M surfactants. It can be seen that in a shampoo containing 10–20% sodium lauryl sulfate, most of the detergent (98–99%) is present in the form of micelles. Even if the shampoo is diluted tenfold upon application to wet hair, as much as 88% of the surfactant is still in the form of micellular aggregates. The possibility exists, therefore, that solubilization is a major factor in shampoo cleaning.

As with rollback, soil removal by solubilization is greatly increased through rubbing and flexing of hair (mechanical work) and increasing temperature. More work needs to be done to precisely determine the contribution of solubilization in the hair-cleaning process.

Emulsification, Penetration, and Mesophase Formation

Emulsification and mesophase, or liquid crystal, formation are two important mechanisms that can be involved in removal of soil from hair. Emulsification involves the breaking down of an oily soil into smaller particles that can form a stable suspension. It requires a low interfacial tension between the oily soil and the bath medium, which may be accomplished by adsorption of shampoo surfactant onto the soil surface. Mechanical work also helps in breaking up of the soil.

Amphiphilic compounds in soils, such as fatty alcohols or fatty acids, can greatly aid the emulsification process by interacting with the shampoo detergent to spontaneously emulsify the soil. Since the shampooing process is short, emulsified soils need be suspended for only a few moments.

Phase diagrams of detergents, water, and certain polar salts such as fatty acids and alcohols can contain large regions that flow easily and are composed of a liquid crystalline phase. Such mesophase formation with amphiphiles, or oily soils containing amphiphiles, constitutes another important mechanism for soil removal from hair.

6.10.9 EFFICACY OF SOIL REMOVAL BY SHAMPOOS

The soils most commonly found on hair originate from three sources: secretions from the body, residues from hair care products, and deposits from the environment. The first type of soil is composed mostly of sebum from the sebaceous glands. Residues from hair care products include hairspray resins and various conditioning materials, while environmental soils include particulate matter from soot, clays, rubber from automobile tires, and so forth.

The efficiency of shampoos in removing these soils and the types of mechanisms by which such removal is carried out depend on a number of factors, including the nature of the soil, the state and condition of the hair surface, and the particular surfactant or combination of surfactants employed in the shampoo. In the following sections the principles of cleaning of different soils by shampoos will be discussed.

6.10.10 CLEANING OF SEBUM

Sebum is probably the single most important soil found on human hair. It is composed of a mixture of lipid materials that are secreted into the follicular duct by the sebaceous glands. The emerging terminal scalp hair is coated with sebum, and mechanical actions such as combing and rubbing against pillows ensure that the sebum becomes distributed more or less evenly over the entire hair surface.

Sebum, which is almost completely molten at body temperature, lubricates the hair, giving it (when not present in excess) a smooth, moisturized feel. Hair with too much sebum on the surface, however, becomes limp and clumped together and is perceived by consumers as dull, dirty, and greasy. Moreover, because it is sticky, the presence of sebum leads to further soiling as a result of adhesion of airborne particulates and other material with which it comes in contact. In addition, sebum can act as a binder, cementing many soil particles together.

Detergents do not penetrate hair appreciably during the relatively short times involved in shampooing. As a result, cleaning of soils such as sebum by shampoos is confined primarily to the hair surface. Internal lipids, however, do not appear to contribute to consumer-perceivable soiling effects. Thus Robbins found that the same quantity of internal lipid (as much as 9% of the total hair weight) could be extracted from both oily and dry hair, indicating that the oily feel of the hair was entirely due to surface sebum. Because of its composition and physical state, sebum can potentially be cleaned from hair by any of the cleaning mechanisms presented in the previous sections. Sebum can be removed from hair by a rollback mechanism. Sebum is also subject to removal by emulsification and mesophase formation. Finally, since the concentrations of surfactants during cleaning are generally well above the surfactant CMCs, sebum can also be cleaned from hair by solubilization.

The relative importance of these mechanisms in cleaning sebum from hair is not identical and more than one cleaning mechanism can certainly operate simultaneously. In any case, the multiplicity of possible cleaning mechanisms for sebum might lead one to expect that shampoos would be very effective in removing sebum from hair. This expectation is supported by much of the literature: a number of studies have demonstrated that anionic surfactants at normal shampoo concentrations can clean surface lipids effectively. Effective cleaning of lipids by anionic surfactants was also reported, and gas-chromatographic techniques were used to measure percent removal from hair of the various components of an artificial sebum. Table 29.2 lists some of the results from this work. It can be seen that the more polar fractions of the sebum, such as free fatty acids, were removed from hair to a greater extent than the less polar fractions, such as paraffin. In other words, hydrophobic soils, like paraffin, have a greater affinity for the hydrophobic hair surface than do more polar deposits and are therefore more difficult to remove.

Sodium laureth-2 sulfate (SLES-2) is seen in Table 29.2 to remove sebum fractions from hair more effectively than ammonium lauryl sulfate (ALS). One reason for this may be related to higher adsorption of SLES-2 than of SLS, which would favor increased removal of sebum by the rollback mechanism.

Table 29.2. Sebum Cleaning by Surfactants

Sebum Component	% Removal by SLES-2	% Removal by ALS
Triglycerides	94.7	94.6
Free fatty acids	96.2	97.1
Spermaceti wax	96.2	84.6
Squalene	98.4	87.6
Paraffin	95.2	80.8
Average % removal	**95.9**	**85.9**

Source: Reference [3]

6.10.11 CLEANING OF QUATERNARY AMMONIUM COMPOUNDS

Conditioners are used to increase ease of hair combing, reduce flyaway, and improve the feel of the hair. The most widely used conditioning agents in commercial products are quaternary ammonium compounds. These compounds are generally used in combination with lipid conditioners such as long-chain alcohols.

Two of the most widely used quaternary conditioners are stearalkonium chloride (SAC) and cetrimonium chloride (CTAC). Other important quats include steartrimonium chloride, dicetydimonium chloride, and tricetylmonium chloride. The most important lipid conditioners include cetyl and stearyl alcohols. Concentrations of cationic surfactants in commercial conditioners are generally on the order of 1–2%, while lipid concentrations are equal to or greater than those of the quats.

Conditioners are generally used at pH levels above the isoelectric point of hair, that is, on negatively charged fiber surfaces. Quaternary ammonium compounds, by virtue of their positive charge, are therefore substantive to the hair surface. Treating hair with these compounds results in a hydrophobic coating that is soft and easy to comb. The binding to hair of quaternary compounds has been found to increase with increases in the hydrophobic chain length and number of chains. This hydrophobic dependence indicates that van der Waals forces play an important role in the deposition of quats on hair.

Deposition of quaternary conditioners on hair is also a function of the degree of negative charge on the hair surface. Compared to virgin hair, bleached hair, which has a more negatively charged surface, retains more than twice the amount of stearalkonium chloride.

Table 29.3. Detergent Cleaning of Stearalkonium Chloride

Treatment	SAC (mg)/g Wool	Detergent (mg)/g Wool
1% SAC	6.68	--
5% ALS	--	1.94
1% SAC/5% ALS	4.58	4.09
5% SDES-2	--	1.94
1% SAC/5% SDES-2	2.52	2.12

Source: Reference [3]

Many quats deposited from conditioning products have been reported to build up over time, indicating that removal of these materials from hair may be more difficult than is the case for sebum. One reason for this is simply the strong electrostatic attraction between the positively charged quats and the negatively charged hair surface. Another reason is that, since quaternary ammonium conditioners are solids, they are not subject to removal by the rollback mechanism. In addition, the positive charge on quats interferes with the mechanism for particulate soil removal, that is, the introduction of negative potentials on soil and substrate as a result of adsorption of anionic surfactant.

Solubilization is a possible mechanism for cleaning of quaternary conditioners. Reich and coworkers have shown, however, that, at least for SAC and CTAC, solubilization by lauryl and laureth sulfates is ineffective. Instead, cleaning with these surfactants results in the formation of insoluble surfactant:quat complexes that are dulling and difficult to remove from hair.

Reducing the hydrophobic chain length of the cleaning surfactant to ten carbon atoms results in formation of more soluble surfactant:quat complexes, which can be more readily cleaned from the hair. Thus washing deposited SAC with 5% sodium deceth-2 sulfate (SDES-2) resulted in higher removal of the deposited conditioner.

The above findings apply to cleaning of the pure quaternary conditioners; cleaning of deposits from fully formulated conditioners lead to improved removal by ALS.

Despite increased quat removal from a fully formulated conditioner, insoluble complex formation between SAC and ALS still occurs. This is evidenced by the increase in deposited ALS measured after cleaning the residue with this surfactant.

6.10.12 CLEANING OF POLYMERIC RESIDUE

Several types of polymers can be found on hair as a result of use of hair care products, including hairspray resins, silicone conditioners, and cationic conditioning polymers. The ease of removal of these polymers from hair depends on several factors, including charge, molecular weight, structure, nature of side chains, and so forth. In the following sections, the ease of cleaning of several important examples of hair care polymers will be discussed.

Cationic Conditioning Polymers

Several cationic polymers are available commercially that provide conditioning benefits, especially increased ease of wet combing. Important examples include polyquaternium 10, a quaternized hydroxyethylcellulose polymer; polyquaternium-11, a copolymer of vinylpyrrolidone and dimethylaminoethyl methacrylate quaternized with dimethyl sulfate; polyquaternium-16, a copolymer of vinylpyrrolidone and quaternized vinylimidazole; polyquaternium-7, a copolymer of diallyldimethylammonium chloride and acrylamide; and polyquaternium-6, a homopolymer of diallyldimethylammonium chloride. As a result of their cationic nature, these conditioning polymers are substantive to hair.

Deposition on hair fibers has been claimed to be an inverse function of charge density, an effect that has been explained by noting that the greater the charge density, the lower the weight of polymer needed to neutralize the total negative charge on the hair.

Polyquaternium-10 is quite substantive to hair, resisting complete removal by SLS even after exposure to detergent for as long as 30 minutes. Similar results were obtained in cleaning experiments with radio-tagged polyquaternium-10. First, as with monofunctional quats, deposition of polyquaternium-10 was found to increase with increasing negative charge on the hair. Thus bleached hair was found to bind more than 2.3 times the amount of polyquat as did untreated hair. In addition, bound polyquaternium-10 was found to be difficult to remove: only 43% of the polyquat could be removed from wool swatches in a single washing with SLS.

Reducing the charge density on the polyquaternium-10 led to more complete cleaning. Thus in a single SLS wash, 75% of this polyquaternium could be removed from wool swatches. Results similar to the above were obtained with polyquaternium-7, which was found to be about as resistant as polyquaternium-10 to removal from wool substrates. The difficulty in cleaning these polymers does not appear to be related to formation of insoluble conditioner:detergent complexes, as was the case with SAC and CTAC. This is evidenced by the fact that cleaning polymer-treated wool with SLS was not observed to result in detergent buildup, even after several cycles of polymer/detergent treatment. It is concluded, therefore, that the difficulty in cleaning polyquats is most likely related to the multiple points of attachment between the polymer and the keratin surface. In order to clean these polymers, it is necessary to break all the points of attachment at the same time, a more difficult proposition than the elimination of the single point of attachment between a small molecule and the hair surface.

Fixative Residue

The holding properties of styling products such as hairsprays, mousses, gels, and setting lotions are provided by various polymeric resins. These materials are generally neutral or negatively charged in order to facilitate removal from hair. Typical examples include the copolymer of vinyl acetate and crotonic acid, the ethyl ester of the copolymer of polyvinyl methyl ether and maleic anhydride (PVM/MA), the copolymer of polyvinyl pyrrolidone and vinyl acetate (PVP/VA), and the copolymer of octylacrylamide/acrylates/butylaminoethyl methacrylate.

The ease of cleaning of hairspray resins was measured using the radio-tagged ethyl ester of PVM/MA. A single washing with 10% SLS resulted in removal of 89%

of the deposited resin. This is also consistent with the expectation that noncationic fixatives would be easier to remove from hair than positively charged polymers.

Dimethicone Residue

As was stated in the introduction, the active ingredient in most two-in-one shampoos is dimethicone, a hydrophobic polymer (polydimethylsiloxane), which is commonly found in many conditioners.

As was the case with fixative resins, little has been published in the literature on the ease of removal of dimethicone. One quantitative study, however, was performed by Rushton and coworkers, who used electronic spectrum for chemical analysis (ESCA) and atomic absorption measurements to study buildup and cleaning of dimethicone. ESCA measurements by Rushton indicated a dimethicone buildup of roughly 35% after five washings of virgin hair with a commercial two-in-one shampoo. After five washings, however, no further buildup was observed. In addition, Rushton found that more than 90% of deposited dimethicone could be removed by a single wash with a commercial shampoo.

6.10.13 EFFECT OF SHAMPOOS ON HAIR

The immediately preceding sections dealt with cleaning of soils by shampoos. Shampoos are also involved in damage of hair, either directly, through removal of structural components of the hair fiber, or indirectly, through removal of protective deposits on the hair. These processes are discussed in the following sections.

Direct Damage by Shampoos

Studies in the literature have indicated that the nonkeratinous regions of the hair, which include the endocuticle, or inner portion of the cuticle, and the cell membrane complex are susceptible to damage by surfactant molecules.

These and additional experiments indicate that exposure to shampoos can have a deleterious effect on hair structure over time. The extent and consequences of these effects are unclear, especially since preexisting damage may render the hair more susceptible to surfactant damage.

Indirect Damage by Shampoos

The use of shampoos can damage hair indirectly as a result of fiber abrasion occurring when hairs are rubbed against each other during cleaning. More important to the damage process, however, is the removal of sebum from the fiber surface during shampooing. This is because sebum acts as a natural lubricant for hair; removal of this material increases damage from grooming, due to chipping, fragmenting, and tearing away of cuticle cells, and it should be attributed to combing and brushing.

Figure 29.1 shows an example of the damage than can occur from grooming. This rather extreme example was induced by washing a tress of virgin hair with a cleaning shampoo and then combing it 700 times while wet. It can be seen that cuticle damage is widespread, with noticeable loss of some cuticle cells and extensive lifting of others from the hair surface. Repeated grooming of the hair gradually erodes the cuticle cells, with the greatest loss occurring at the tips of the hair. Eventually all of the cuticle cells can be lost, exposing the cortex and resulting in a split end. An example of such splitting is shown in Figure 29.2.

Damage to Chemically Treated Hair

Permanent waving, bleaching, and oxidative dyeing can result in significant damage to the hair. In addition to causing tensile damage, all of these treatments oxidize the surface of the hair, resulting in a considerable increase in surface friction. This subjects the hair to increased grooming damage because sebum is easier to clean from an oxidized hair surface, while combing forces are increased as a result of increased friction.

Chemically treated hair is also subject to increased water swelling and penetration by different materials as a result of reduced disulfide cross-linking and damage to nonkeratinous regions of the hair, including the cell membrane complex. Increased uptake of surfactants can, of course, lead to direct damage as a result of increased extraction of structural components of the hair fiber.

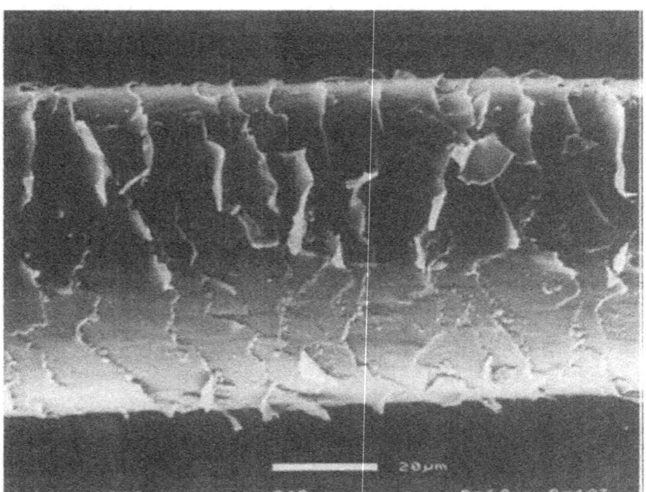

Figure 29.1. Combing damage resulting from washing a hair tress with a cleaning shampoo and then combing 700 times while wet. The scanning electron micrograph (SEM) is typical of hair taken from the combed tress. Note raised and chipped cuticle cells, and areas where cells have been completely torn away.

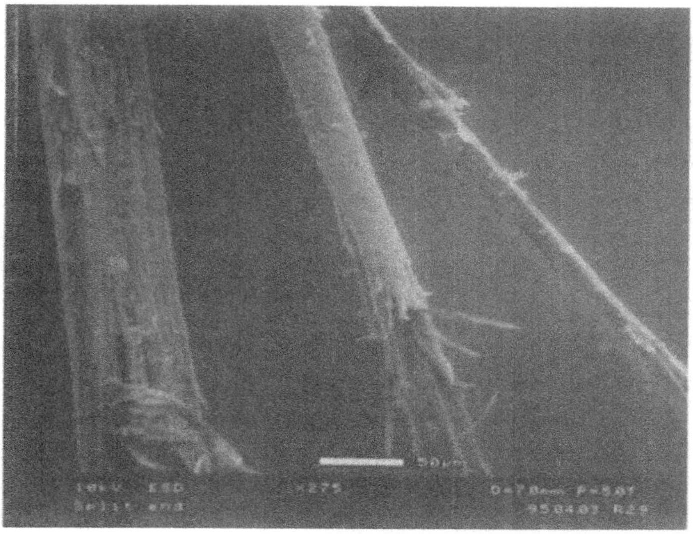

Figure 29.2. SEM photograph of a split end. Note the structure in the exposed cortex.

SECTION III: SHAMPOO EVALUATION

Formula Evaluation

Along with testing on actual hair, the shampoo formula itself needs to be tested for certain attributes. One of the most important tests a formula must make it through is shelf stability. Accelerated testing in different temperature/humidity extremes is usually used to evaluate the stability of a formula. Foam height and density is another very important attribute, but before it is tested on tresses, the actual foam height needs to be measured. The last formula attribute that needs to be taken into consideration is the ease of manufacturing. If the formula is not scalable, it is not marketable.

Stability

Products going on the store shelves should have at least two years of shelf life. During this time period, the shampoo should not see appreciable changes in viscosity, color, or fragrance. Multiphase products should not separate and there should be no precipitation seen.

Accelerated aging tests are run to test product stability. These tests are usually run at temperature extremes to simulate warehouse storage or shipping conditions. There are no standard accelerated aging tests for hair care products, so most manufacturers develop their own. A typical shampoo accelerated aging test suggests oven storage at 40°C and 50°C for three to six months as well as 25°C for a year.

Samples should be packaged in glass as well as the packaging that the shampoo would be sold in. The products should also go through one or more freeze/thaw cycles to evaluate the effects of lower temperatures [2].

Foam Height/Density

Foam is a very important attribute of a shampoo. Consumers will evaluate a shampoo based on the quality and quantity of the foam produced even though most shampoos have much more surfactant in them than actually needed to clean the hair. Strong abundant foam is directly related to the cleaning mechanism of a shampoo according to the average consumer.

There are various tests to measure the foaming potential of shampoos in the absence and presence of lipids. One very simple test is by shaking a known concentration of the shampoo formula in a graduated cylinder for a set amount of time. The foam height is then measured after shaking.

Manufacturing Ease

When formulating a shampoo, the ease in which it is manufactured or scaled up must be taken into consideration. A complex formula opens up more opportunity for production error. Order of addition, viscosity adjustments, mixing equipment, as well as heating capacity all need to be thought out carefully when transferring a formula from lab or pilot scale to manufacturing scale.

Evaluation of Shampoo Performance

A stable formulation is just the beginning for a shampoo formulator; performance of the shampoo ties together the entire gamete of consumer-driven traits that a formula must exhibit. These can be tested in a laboratory on tresses and if all goes well, the formulas can be tested by trained cosmetologists using half-head test methodology. This type of testing does not involve consumer evaluation, but is useful because it eliminates the differences seen in various hair types. Finally, once the shampoo passes all laboratory and half-head testing, it can move on to consumer testing. This is usually carried out in salons or at cosmetology schools with salons. Only after consumer approval for efficacy and safety, should the formulas go to market.

The following sections introduce some of the important attributes that are looked at when evaluating a shampoo's performance.

Ease of Application

This attribute is related to shampoo viscosity. A shampoo should be viscous enough to remain in the palm of the hand during pouring, but should easily disperse over the hair during application.

Lather

It is important for the foam height of the shampoo to be checked before it is added to hair, but the lather needs to be evaluated on tresses also. This should take into consideration the speed and amount of lather generated, the quality as well as the stability on hair. An extension of lather generation is lather rinsability. Water hardness, temperature, and rinsing rate all need to be taken into account when rinsing is evaluated, as well as any residuals left on the hair once rinsing is complete.

Wet/Dry Comb

Combing ease can be defined as the ease of aligning hair fibers in a parallel arrangement with a comb. Evaluations of combing ease, especially on wet hair, are often used as the primary assessment for the broader consumer attribute of hair conditioning, which also includes hair softness and lubricity. Hair fiber properties that improve combing ease are increasing stiffness, diameter, and cohesion; and decreasing curvature, friction, length, and static charge. Studies have indicated how different types of hair treatments can affect combing ease. Shampoos can affect several of these properties depending on the particular formulation. For instance, high-cleaning shampoos can make the hair more difficult to comb by removing sebum and oily soils that can lubricate the hair, while conditioning shampoos can deposit materials on the hair that decrease friction and thereby make the hair easier to comb [3].

The ease of combing attribute includes ease of snag removal and ease of comb slip on both wet and dry hair. Methods to evaluate combing ease include both qualitative combing of tresses combined with statistical evaluation of the results and quantitative instrumental methods. Instrumental methods involve the measurement of combing forces on tresses following treatment using an Instron or Diastron tensile tester [3].

Luster/Shine

Luster or shine is a very important aesthetic property to the consumer. Aging hair, chemical treatments, buildup of styling products, use of heated styling tools, as well as certain shampoo ingredients can all add to the dulling process. Shampoos that claim to add shine have a great market advantage as consumers associate this added shine or luster to creating healthy strong hair.

There are many instrumental methods as well as subjective evaluations that can be used to evaluate shine or luster on hair. No matter which method is employed, there are several factors that need to be taken into consideration when substantiating a claim for luster or shine enhancement: fiber straightness, degree of alignment of the hair, as well as hair color.

Volume/Body

The consumer attribute of body is both a visual and a tactile hair property indicative of fullness and volume combined with springiness and bounce. The effects shampoos have on hair body are formula dependent. For instance, deep-cleaning shampoos containing higher amounts of anionic surfactants can provide an increase in body by removing surface oils that weigh down hair. These types of shampoos can be marketed as volumizing or shampoos for fine/thin hair. Alternatively, shampoos containing materials than can build up on the hair can reduce hair body [3].

Several instrumental methods have been developed to evaluate parameters associated with hair body. These approaches measure changes in fiber friction, stiffness, curvature, diameter, weight, cohesion, and length. Treatments that increase the hair's curvature or diameter increase the frictional forces between fibers, or make the hair stiffer will increase body; those that increase the cohesion between fibers or weigh them down will decrease hair body [3].

Manageability

Manageability is a measure of styling ease and style retention. It is a complex consumer attribute that is difficult to assess by any one hair parameter or method. It has been suggested that evaluators consider three types of manageability: style arrangement manageability, style retention manageability, and flyaway manageability (static control). These properties can be assessed best by using a control treatment. As with other attributes, the effects that a particular shampoo has on manageability can vary. Any assessment of manageability is further complicated by factors involving the type of hair, humidity, and style [3].

Fragrance

Fragrance may not be a performance attribute for a shampoo formulation, but its importance cannot be overlooked. The effects that fragrance can have on a shampoo go far beyond that of formulation compatibility. The lasting power and acceptability of a fragrance needs to be taken into consideration before a formulation goes to market.

SECTION IV: FUTURE TRENDS IN SHAMPOOS

Consumer demand directs the mainstream shampoo market, which is why it is important for the formulator to stay abreast of any upcoming or lasting trends.

Natural and Biodegradable Ingredients

As stated before, consumers are becoming more aware of what they are putting on their bodies, as well as what is being done to the environment. Consumers perceive natural or naturally derived ingredients to be milder and safer than their synthetic counterparts as well as more eco-friendly. Ingredients that have chemical-sounding names are usually not deemed natural by the average consumer, so cosmetics and personal care items are trending more toward naturally derived ingredients and simplicity on the label. The biggest problem plaguing the formulator is that natural ingredients are sometimes hard to work with and don't necessarily function the same as the synthetic or chemically modified ingredients. Yet the consumer expects the natural shampoo to have the same attributes as a regular shampoo.

Many shampoo manufacturers have come out with "natural" product lines. These formulations may not be all-natural, but many contain biodegradable surfactants as well as botanicals and oils to replace some of the synthetic ingredients used in their regular formulas.

Anti-Aging Benefits

It is no secret that the anti-aging trend has taken over the cosmetic world. Staying young, or at least the perception of staying young, has spilled over into the hair care industry. As hair gets older, it gets coarser, the color fades; it becomes thinner and loses some of its natural luster. Shampoos are being manufactured that have anti-aging benefits that claim to help combat some of the issues hair goes through as it ages.

The "Free" Shampoo

Whether it be sulfate-free, amide-free, paraben-free, or silicone-free, there will always be the consumer demand for some type of "free" shampoo. These trends cycle and depend highly upon which ingredient is the hot topic of the moment. Even though the type of "free" shampoo can have a short life span and are of the specialty type, these shampoos have made it from being seen only in salons, to the mainstream store shelves.

Dry Shampoos

Although not necessarily a shampoo in conventional terms, the dry shampoo, once popular in the 1970s, is making a strong comeback, especially in European countries. This type of shampoo is not only brought back for its convenience factor, but also to satisfy the growing number of people who worry about the consequences of shampooing every day.

Dry shampoos are simple formulas consisting primarily of a corn or rice starch, which is used to absorb oils from the scalp and hair. Most modern dry shampoos also contain some sort of conditioning agent so that they don't leave the hair stiff like the very first formulas did. The problem facing this type of "shampoo" is that the starch used for these shampoos is white, so it is not very adequate for use in very dark hair.

REFERENCES

1. Mirajkar, Yelloji-Rao K., Application of Surfactants in Shampoos, Chapter 8 in *Handbook of Detergents*, Zoller, Uri ed., CRC Press, 2008, 151–180
2. Tarng, Jiashi J. and Reich, Charles, Shampoos and Conditioners, Chapter 10 in *Liquid Detergents*, Lai, Kuo Yann, ed., CRC Press, Boca Raton, FL, 2005. 377–449.
3. Reich C and J Chupa, Hair Shampoos, Chapter 29 in *Harry's Cosmeticology, 8th Edition*, Reiger, M. ed., Chemical Publishing Company, New York, 2000.
4. Wong, Michael, Cleansing of Hair, Chapter 3 in *Hair and Hair Care*, Johnson, Dale H., ed., Marcel Dekker, Inc., New York, 1997.
5. Panda, H., Cosmetics for The Hair, Chapter 6 in *Herbal Cosmetics Handbook*, Asia Pacific Business Press, Delhi, India, 2004.
6. Dalrymple, Damon M., Tommey, Ann B., Kortemeier, Uta, Multifunctional Ingredients in Hair Care Products, Chapter 3 in *Multifunctional Cosmetics*, Schueller, Randy and Romanowski, Perry, ed., Marcel Dekker, Inc, New York, 2001.
7. Steinberg, David C., Common Preservatives, Chapter 2 in *Preservatives for Cosmetics: Second Edition,* Allured Publishing Corporation, Carol Stream, IL, 2006.
8. A course on Hair Care Technology Symposium, Instructed by Colleen Rocafort, Joseph Dallal and John Bozza. Presented on August 24–26, 2010. Glenpointe Marriott, Teaneck, NJ.
9. Romanowski, Perry, Why does salt thicken Shampoo?, www.chemistcorner.com/why-does-salt-thicken-shampoo/.
10. Schueller, Randy and Romanowski, Perry, *Beginning Cosmetic Chemistry,* second edition, Allured Publishing Corporation, Carol Stream, IL, 2003, 217–226.
11. Clarke, Mary T., Rheological Additives, Chapter 4 in *Rheological Properties of Cosmetics and Toiletries*, Laba, Dennis, ed., Marcel Dekker, Inc, New York, 1993.
12. Hossain, Md. Mohsin, Interactions Between Starch and Surfactants by Ternary Phase Diagram, *Canadian Journal on Scientific and Industrial Research*, May 2012, Vol. 3, No. 4, 246–253.
13. Kozlowski, Angela C., Formulary in *Cosmetic and Toiletries Hair Care: From Physiology to Formulation*, Allured Publishing Corporation, Carol Stream, IL 2008, pg 556, 559.

GLOSSARY

viscosity – thickness of a liquid or resistance to flow.

rheology – the study of the flow of liquids.

anionic – negatively charged ion.

nonionic – does not have a positive or negative charge.

cationic – positively charged ion.

amphoteric – can act as a positive or negative ion depending upon pH.

zwitterionic – ion with both positive and negative charge attached to the same molecule with an overall neutral charge but can act as either a positive or a negative depending on pH.

flash foam – foam that develops immediately, may not have lasting power.

emulsifier – substance that stabilizes an emulsion by keeping both the water and oil phases mixed.

cloud point – point at which dissolved solids are no longer completely soluble, causing a solution to appear cloudy.

hydrophilic – has an affinity for water.

hydrophobic – repels water.

micelle – an aggregate of molecules that form in colloidal solutions.

pseudoplastic rheology – also known as sheer thinning. Viscosity will thin upon movement.

substantive – will bind to a substrate (hair) and not wash off with normal washing.

dent corn – a common variety of corn that has a ratio of about 76% amylopectin and 24% amylose. Used for making corn starches.

waxy corn – a variant of corn that contains 100% amylopectin. Used for making corn starches, not as common as dent corn.

amylopectin – a branched polysaccharide with α-1,4 and α-1,6 linkages. Makes up 76% of dent corn starch and 100% of waxy corn starch.

amylose – a linear polysaccharide with α-1,4 linkages. Makes up 24% of dent corn starch.

gelatinization temperature – the temperature at which a starch begins to swell.

antioxidant – substance that counteracts the damaging effects of oxidation.

sequestrant – form chelate compounds with metal ions often found in hard water. This allows for a shampoo to be rinsed easily from the hair without forming a layer of "scum" on the hair.

humectant – a substance that retains moisture.

critical micelle concentration (CMC) – concentration of surfactant above which micelles form and all additional surfactants added will spontaneously form micelles.

sebum – an oily secretion of the sebaceous gland that can be found on the scalp.

PART 6.11

HAIR STYLING

Author
Charles Warren

a. Nonpressurized Styling Products

b. Pressurized Styling Products

The art of styling hair requires a broad spectrum of products to help achieve and maintain the desired coiffure. These products vary from those intended to simply hold hair in place (finishing products) to those intended to actually build a desired style (working products). A professional stylist would say that all styling is related to either lifting hair up or holding hair down. Styles can be achieved chemically by permanent waves or straighteners, mechanically by rollers, or thermally by irons or any combination of the former. In the development and maintenance of the desired configuration, a wide range of styling products may be used.

The styling product category is the largest and most confusing of all of the categories to the consumer. The formulator needs to understand what the product is to be used for in order to develop the best formula for the intended product. Once the targeted consumer and the desired functionality is understood, the formulator can develop the required formula and form to deliver the intended result in an aesthetically pleasing form.

In general, styling products can be separated into two categories: non-aerosolized styling products and pressurized aerosol styling products. Non-aerosolized styling products can be categorized into liquids, gels, nonpressurized sprays, and specialized (e.g., waxes, hairdressings) styling products. Pressurized aerosolized products can be categorized as fixatives (e.g., hairsprays/mousses) or specialty (e.g., shine sprays) products.

Because of the nature of styling products—the basic formulations and usage platforms—they are the most highly regulated category in hair care. The formulator needs to be aware of all of the regulatory requirements by category in order to develop functional, compliant formulations. The Volatile Organic Compound (VOC) regulations on styling products exist at the federal level (EPA) and at individual state levels, California being one of the strictest. Because the regulatory environment is dynamic and new interpretations arise on an almost daily basis, great diligence is required in formulating and even naming products in this category. The formulator must work closely with legal and regulatory advisors to avoid inadvertently developing a formula that will later be declared noncompliant and subject to punitive legal issues.

a. Nonpressurized Styling Products

Liquids and Gels

In general, both of these subcategories fulfill similar functions—to develop a style and then, once dry, maintain that desired configuration. Styling liquids are water-thin, aqueous, or hydro-alcoholic solutions of a holding, film-forming polymer (e.g., PVP and/or derivatives), modifiers to increase plasticity (i.e., flexibility) of dried film, and aesthetic modifiers (e.g., fragrance). They are generally applied to damp hair, worked through the hair, then dried after the desired configuration is achieved. They can be used in combination with brushing while blow-drying to achieve volume/fullness, which will be maintained as the film dries on the individual hairs.

Styling gels serve a similar function, but applied in a gel form. The gel itself is formed by the use of a polymeric material (e.g., carbomer) and provides a thicker coating to the individual hairs. Gels may be used to hold hair in a flat configuration or in conjunction with brushing and blow-drying to achieve volume or raise hair from the scalp.

When liquids or gels dry they form a film on the hairs and cause the hairs to hold together in a relatively rigid configuration. If combed or manipulated after drying, this film coating and the resultant "welding" of hairs together is disrupted and will no longer hold. This disruption can be negative if the desired configuration was achieved or positive if the desired configuration is less rigid and will be supplemented with other fixative products. Regardless, as the film is disrupted it breaks into small particles that can manifest themselves as flakes or dust. The formulator can incorporate materials to ameliorate this negative appearance, but must certainly be aware of the potential for this occurring.

Nonpressurized Aerosol Sprays

These sprays are hydro-alcoholic solutions of a hair-fixative polymer or polymers, film modifiers, and aesthetic materials. They are sprayed directly onto damp (working sprays) or dry (fixative) hair. They provide a modicum of coating to the individual hair fibers (used as working spray) or "spot welds" at the junction of individual hairs (used as fixative spray).

When used as a working product, these function in a similar fashion to liquids and gels, but allow lower levels of product to be applied. As a finishing product, these sprays dispense a fine coating of fixative polymer on the final coiffure to help maintain the desired configuration. Dispensing water or hydro-alcoholic solution onto dry hair will disrupt the hydrogen bonds of the hair and can cause the desired configuration to collapse or be disrupted. The formulator needs to be aware of how the product can disrupt a coiffure and can select a sprayer that, in conjunction with the degree of hold required (i.e., the amount of fixative polymer delivered to the hair), will ameliorate this collapse or disruption.

b. Pressurized Styling Products

Aerosol Hairsprays

Pressurized styling products (e.g., hairsprays and mousse) have been and are the largest section of the styling products universe and, combined with gels, comprise between 80–90% of the entire styling category.

Formulating pressurized hairsprays requires technical understanding of the basic formulas and mechanical understanding of the way that pressurized aerosols work and, specifically, how the formula, propellant, and spray button/valve system interact to deliver the desired outcome. In this particular subcategory, all of the parts make up the "formula," and changing any of the parts will have s significant impact on the final product. In addition, this category is highly impacted by the VOC regulations mentioned earlier.

The base formula for hairsprays is essentially an alcoholic or hydroalcoholic solution containing a polymeric resin or resins (fixatives), a neutralizing agent (if required by resin type), plasticizing agents to impact the stiffness/brittleness of the dried film, fragrance, and claims ingredients. The propellants used for hairsprays are propane, butane, isobutane, and in the world of VOC regulation, hydrofluorocarbon 152a.

The ratio of base formula to propellant (base-prop ratio) is important for product performance. In general, the lower the base-prop ratio, the finer and dryer the resulting spray.

In general, the volatile organic compounds in a pressurized aerosol hairspray are the alcohol (solvent for the base) and the hydrocarbon propellants. To achieve the requisite VOC maximum, the formulator would commonly use: a) a combination of alcohol, water, dimethylether (DME—a solvent/propellant that ameliorates propellant/base miscibility but is a VOC), and hydrocarbon; or, b) a combination of alcohol, hydrocarbon, and hydrofluorocarbon 152a. In the DME/water approach, the water, resins, neutralizing agents, and other miscellaneous ingredients are the non-VOC portion; the propellant, DME, and alcohol are the VOCs, which have a maximum level allowable. In the 152a approach, the resins, neutralizing agents, and other miscellaneous ingredients are the non-VOC portion; the propellant, 152a, and alcohol are the VOCs, which have a maximum level allowable. There are some special exemption formulations that have been used for compliance, but the two approaches indicated are the most common.

Water-containing hairsprays tend to be "wetter" when applied, and water can negatively impact coiffures, can cause corrosion in electro-tinplated steel cans and valves (commonly used for hairsprays), and can require special gaskets not negatively impacted by DME. The use of water in the hairspray can make the formula less expensive than the 152a approach. The 152a approach yields a finer, drier spray, does not impact the final coiffure, and is not corrosive to valves and cans. However, the 152a approach is significantly more expensive.

Mousse

Mousse styling products are used for a combination of styling and hair holding. In general, mousse formulations are an aqueous solution of holding resins (e.g., VP/VA copolymer), conditioners (e.g., polyquaternium-4, dimethicone copolyol), surfactant materials (e.g., polysorbate 60), aesthetic/claims ingredients (e.g., fragrance), and propellant (e.g., butane, propane, and isoubutane). When properly formulated, the propellant phase becomes dispersed in the liquid base phase such that when dispensed, the product immediately forms a thick foam in the hand, which can then be applied to wet or dry hair for styling. Some mousse formulations contain alcohol to assist the mixing of the water phase and the propellant phase.

Mousse formulations are generally used for a conditioning hold, with the ratio of holding resin and conditioners being varied to provide more or less of the desired property. These products are generally used as the preliminary styling product to create volume or create desired coiffure. They are then followed by a finishing spray to hold the configuration in place. They can be used alone to build and maintain style depending on the desired configuration or in conjunction with other styling forms such as gels or gums.

As are all pressurized styling products, mousse formulations are governed by VOC regulations. The levels of VOC allowed for mousse are substantially lower than that for aerosol hairsprays. The VOCs in mousse formulations are the propellant and alcohol, if included in the formula.

Pressurized Shine Sprays

Generally, pressurized shine sprays are an anhydrous solution of lightweight oils and lipoidal materials, fragrance, and propellant. These products are primarily used by consumers with relaxed, African-Caribbean hair to impart shine. Shine sprays are also regulated for VOC content, and the formulator must be aware of the categorization of the oils used before starting. In addition, the ultimate particle size of the dispensed spray must be closely monitored. Too fine a particle size can lead to inhalation of the oily particles, which can result in significant health issues. The formulator needs to check the current regulations.

SPECIALTY STYLING PRODUCTS

Author
Charles Warren

The category of specialty styling products is huge and grows on an almost daily basis. Products are developed to achieve styles and effects. These products usually come from the professional stylist arena and are the result of a creative stylist using an new or alternate material to achieve a particular "look" or style on a particular hair type.

Included in this category are waxes, hairdressings, silicone shine products, gums, etc. These products can all be used to impart a targeted effect on the hair. Waxes and gums are blends of waxes and other higher-molecular-weight fatty materials to impart stiffness to short hair or stiffness to small sections of a larger coiffure—small braids or sideburns for example. Hair dressings are blends of fatty materials or oil/water emulsions or microemulsions used to provide shine, immediate lubrication, and a modicum of control, especially on dry hair. Silicone shine treatments are blends of silicones used to lightly coat the hair and provide a glossy shine.

In general, the formulator needs to know the targeted consumer/hair type, the effect desired, the claims to be made, and the way the product will be used by the consumer to begin formulation work. A survey of the competitive products used for the same purpose will be helpful as a starting point.

PERMANENT WAVING

Author
Charles Warren

Permanent waves are two- or three-component systems applied to hair rolled on appropriate rods to achieve a specific curl or wave pattern that is durable ("permanent"). The first solution is either the waving lotion alone or a two-component system for creating the wave lotion. The waving lotion alone (cold wave) is an aqueous mixture of ammonium hydroxide (1–2% ammonia), thioglycolate (8–10% as thioglycolic acid), surfactant, and other water-soluble ingredients desired. (The pH of a traditional cold wave is 9–9.5.) Ammonium thioglycolate and monoethanolamine thioglycolate are the common forms of thioglycolate employed. It is the thioglycolate ion that is the reactive species. The two-component waving lotion involves an aqueous solution of ammonium hydroxide (1–3% ammonia) to which is added glyceryl monothioglycolate (GMT) immediately prior to application. Again, it is the thioglycolate that is the reactive species. In either case, the waving lotion is applied to the hair wrapped around rods of the appropriate size for the desired curl pattern. The waving lotion is allowed to process under a plastic cap (for the cold wave or some GMT waves) or with a cap under a hot dryer for acid GMT waves) until the desired curl pattern is achieved (determined by the operator unrolling a rod and reviewing a "test curl"). Once the pattern is acceptable, the waving solution is rinsed from the hair and the second component (neutralizer), an aqueous solution of hydrogen peroxide (2–2.5%) is applied to reform the cystine bonds in the new configuration. After five minutes, the neutralizer is rinsed and the rods are removed.

Permanent waves using bisulfate (ammonium or sodium) are also used. These function in a similar fashion to the thioglycolate waves, but have lower negative odor. They are slightly less aggressive on the hair than thioglycolate waves and are subject to a greater degree of reversion to the original hair configuration. Nonetheless, they can be effective on the right hair and with the right expectations.

Permanent waving is moderately damaging to hair due to the alkaline nature of the products and the fact that not all of the cystine bonds that are broken re-form, leaving the hair weaker than prior to the treatment.

PART 6.14

CONDITIONERS/TREATMENTS

Author
Charles Warren

Hair is continually being damaged by mechanical stresses (e.g., combing/brushing), thermal stresses (e.g., blow dryers), and chemical stresses (e.g., coloring/bleaching). As hair has no biological means of repairing itself, the damage is cumulative. Hair grows at a rate of 0.25 to 0.33 inches per month, so hair that is eight inches long (medium length) has undergone 2–2.5 years of cumulative damage. The additional mechanical stress of hair fibers rubbing back and forth across each other (fiber-fiber) interaction is an additional source of damage that is not usually even thought of.

Damaged hair becomes weaker, leads to breakage and fiber splitting, loses cuticle (the flattened outer protective layer of hair), and develops an overall negative surface charge. This negative charge results in "fly-away" hair, appearing frizzy and dull. Damage on the hairs' surface also interferes with the wicking of the natural oils (sebum) secreted at the hair roots, further exacerbating the negative appearance and lubrication of the individual fibers.

Conditioners and treatments serve to neutralize the negative charge on the hairs' surface, restore oil to the fibers' and leave the hair softer and shinier, at least on a temporary basis. Rinses, conditioners, and treatments generally serve the same functions, the difference being the amount and types of materials used. They are all usually oil-in-water emulsions (lipoidal ingredients suspended in a continuous phase of water, held together with emulsifiers). They usually contain a cationic (positively charged moiety) such as stearalkonium or cetrimonium chloride (quaternary ammonium compounds) and a blend of fatty alcohols, such as cetyl or stearyl alcohols. In addition, there are aesthetic ingredients such as fragrance and colors, microbiological preservatives and other conditioning/claims ingredients such as proteins, and vitamins.

Conditioners can be divided into the general categories of leave-in conditioners, rinses, moisturizing conditioners, volumizing conditioners, conditioning treatments, and specialty conditioners, such as oil or protein treatments. Again, there may be multiple names and types of conditioners, but they will usually fit into one of these categories.

The formulator needs to balance the ingredients to maintain a stable emulsion and deliver the end result claimed. Understanding the emulsion and the desired end result is usually a significant challenge and requires technical understanding as well as the ability to interpret all of the aesthetic requirements for the emulsion itself, the manufacture and dispensing of the emulsion, the feel of the product on the hands and hair as applied, and, most importantly, the final appearance and feel of the hair. Not enough conditioning will provide the hair with little benefit and too much conditioning can leave the hair looking/feeling greasy and weighed down. A poor emulsion will result in separation and instability, or if overemulsified, an unpleasant greasy and ineffective formula.

Leave-in conditioners are either water-thin aqueous solutions containing a cationic moiety (usually a cationic polymeric material) to neutralize charge and provide some conditioning to the hair fibers. They are low in lipoidal materials and usually dispensed via a spray directly on the hair or onto the hands and then worked through the hair.

Rinses are thin, rinse-out emulsions applied to the hair post-shampoo and contain lower percentages of cationic materials (quaternary ammonium salts), fatty alcohols, and ancillary or aesthetic ingredients. They provide a lower level of conditioning, desired by some consumers and effective in ameliorating the negative effects of relatively minor damage. As these are relatively thin emulsions, they can be problematic in maintaining stability over time and through extremes of heat and cold.

Moisturizing conditioners are emulsions containing higher levels of both cationic moieties (quaternary ammonium salts, cationic polymers) and lipoidal materials (fatty alcohols and oils). They are rinse-out, post-shampoo treatments and are dispensed into the hand and applied to the hair, left on for an interval, and then rinsed from the hair. They are generally thicker emulsions and have a creamy feel that is aesthetically pleasing to the consumer while being applied and worked through the hair, signaling efficacy while doing the actual conditioning of the hair. These conditioners are effective in neutralizing the negative charge, leaving residual oils on the hair surface and softening the hair fibers—the greater the degree of damage to the hair (and, thus, the porosity or ability for hair to absorb), the higher the degree of tolerance to lipoidal materials. For example, chemically relaxed (straightened) hair will tolerate and require higher levels of oils and conditioning materials than hair that is damaged by simple combing/blow drying. The formulator needs to be aware of the targeted consumer/hair-type when developing a formula. What delivers an effective and aesthetically pleasing level of conditioning and hair-feel to one consumer will be viewed as oily/greasy to another.

Volumizing conditioners will provide conditioning benefits to finer/thinner hair at low levels and will have the added benefit of leaving behind materials (usually polymeric materials) that will attach to the hair electrostatically and thicken the hair, resulting in a fuller-appearing coiffure. These conditioners are generally trickier to formulate, as consumers with fine/thin hair are highly sensitive to materials perceived as weighing the hair down, leaving it looking flatter and appearing oily or greasy. This category of conditioner is probably the smallest of all of the categories.

Specialty conditioner treatments (e.g., oil or protein treatments) are rinse-out, post-shampoo treatments intended to be applied on an infrequent basis and are generally for a specific problem (e.g., severely damaged hair). In general, the formulas contain higher levels of specific ingredients (e.g., fatty materials), are applied and left on for extended periods (1–10 minutes), and may include the use of a plastic covering (cap) or a moist towel. Some specialty treatments require a shampoo step after the treatment to remove any excess oils or conditioning ingredients. Relaxed (straightened), bleached, or extremely fragile or dry hair are the targeted types for these products.

PART 6.15

HAIR COLORANTS AND PROTECTION

Author
Padmaja Prem, Ph.D
Vice President, Research & Development
Combe Incorporated, 1101 Westchester Avenue
White Plains, NY 10604

ABSTRACT

Most permanent hair-coloring technology is based on the 100+ year-old approach of oxidation of *p*-diamines and *p*-aminophenols by hydrogen peroxide at alkaline pH to form an active intermediate. These active intermediates then react inside the hair fiber with couplers that produce colored molecules of varying size depending on the nature of the primary intermediates and couplers. Being bigger, these color molecules are trapped inside the hair fiber, thus providing resistance to removal. Permanent hair color, however, is far from "permanent." Factors such as frequent washing, UV exposure, and heat styling are generally known to cause hair-color fading.

Additionally, hair-coloring process imparts oxidative damage to hair lipids and keratin and disrupts hair cuticle. When the cuticle is disrupted, it becomes fragmented and rough, resulting in less light reflection from the hair surface. The dramatic increase in the use of hair-coloring products and other chemical treatments requires specific products for the care and protection of color as well as the hair that underwent damage due to oxidation of lipids and proteins. Enhancing the protection of color, shine, vibrancy, and overall appearance and conditioning of color-treated hair requires products that are formulated differently from regular hair care products. Color- and shine-protecting products contain substances that smooth down the cuticle and increase light reflection.

This chapter describes the fundamentals of permanent hair coloring, the change in hair properties associated with hair coloring, and the factors that influence color fading, vibrancy, and shine. Further, it also covers formulation techniques to deliver long-lasting color, color vibrancy, and shine and remedies for protection of color-treated hair to preserved color vibrancy and shine. Beyond these approaches, the author has also provided a unique and critical review of selected ingredients and products in the market offering various benefits for color-treated hair.

The underlying reasons and remedies for hair-color protection described in this chapter provide important leads to ingredient-seekers and product formulators for color care and presents an opportunity for a myriad of novel products that consumers long for. The chapter is also unique in that it provides thoughtful, practical recommendations for developing better hair color and hair care products to address the needs of color-treated hair. This wisdom goes beyond the traditional approach of finding new ingredients or formulations to achieve the goals of beautiful hair that is shiny and vibrant. It is recommended that these approaches be incorporated in literature by product manufacturers as important information to consumers.

TABLE OF CONTENTS

6.15.1 INTRODUCTION

Hair-coloring products are a multibillion-dollar international industry composed of three types of products: temporary, semi-permanent, and permanent hair-color products. The majority of its growth (~70%) is derived from permanent hair-coloring products, which owe their popularity to their long-lasting effect, ease of application, natural look, versatility, and allowing virtually any color to be achieved.[1] This industry is poised for even greater growth in the future due to an increasingly aging, and thus graying, global population longing for a youthful appearance. Permanent coloring technology, which is also called lift and deposit technology, has the ability to lift the natural color of hair and deposit new color that lasts until the hair is replaced by new growth. Most permanent hair-coloring technology is based on the 100+ year-old approach of oxidation of colorless p-diamines and p-aminophenols by hydrogen peroxide at alkaline pH to form active intermediates. Permanent hair colorants are normally marketed in the form of a two-component kit comprising an alkaline composition of oxidation hair dyes in a liquid, gel, or cream vehicle and a developer composition that utilizes an oxidizing agent, usually hydrogen peroxide. The two compositions are mixed immediately prior to application to the hair. The alkaline pH of the resultant mixture causes the hair shaft to swell, allowing the dye precursors to penetrate into the cortex of the hair. These dye precursors are then oxidized and combine to form larger molecules. These larger molecules contain a significant level of conjugated double bonds, hence producing a colored product that is visible from the exterior of the hair. After an appropriate development time during which the composition resides on the hair, the mixture is rinsed from the hair. The color of the hair is then permanently altered.

Permanent hair color, however, is far from "permanent" due to color fading by factors such as frequent washing, light exposure, and other daily grooming habits such as heat styling. Permanent hair coloring changes hair structure due to removal of soluble lipids and oxidation of keratin protein and lipids. These changes in hair structure make colored hair to be more porous than virgin hair. As hair becomes more porous, it absorbs more color and it also removes more color on washing. The fading of permanent hair color due to frequent washing, daily grooming, and by environmental factors has become a common problem of color-treated hair and a source of frequent complaints by consumers.

Photo damage to the hair shaft contributes to dullness by altering the chemistry of the dyed hair through oxidative damage. UV exposure affects hair strength and elasticity and cause photo-oxidation, which triggers discoloration and fading in both natural and color-treated hair. Work by Ph. Maillan reports the use of a leave-on formulation with a polymeric organosiloxane sunscreen to protect the artificially colored hair. This polymeric filter was reported to be more effective than classic sunscreen ethylhexyl methoxycinnamate.

Luster or shine is another important feature of hair's appearance, and this visual effect is a key objective in the consumer hair care market. Thus, shine-protecting hair care products are worthwhile for the consumer with color-treated hair demanding youthful hair appearance. Color strength or color vibrancy is another important attribute for colored hair, but no parameter or test method has previously been developed to combine the two and enable quantified vibrancy claims. In relation, based on work by Lefaudeux et al., the authors define a new parameter for such claims, the hair-color vibrance factor (HCVF).

6.15.2 FUNDAMENTALS OF HAIR COLORING

Hair dyes can be divided mainly into three categories, each with a specific composition and action mechanism: temporary dyes (water-soluble dyes that withstand only one-time shampooing), semi-permanent dyes (which can withstand four to five shampooings), and permanent or oxidative dyes that needs reapplication only when new roots are shown. Temporary hair color works on the surface of hair to add sheer color and it typically only lasts one to two shampoos. When applied to prelightened or extremely porous hair, temporary hair color may penetrate further into the cortex and stain the hair shaft.

Semi-permanent hair color works on the surface of hair to deposit color, yet lasts longer than temporary hair color. Semi-permanent contains large and small color molecules that adhere to the outside of the hair, while some penetrate the cuticle layer, depending on the hair's porosity. Some color is removed with each shampoo, but color typically lasts from four to eight shampoos.

Oxidative hair dyes are the most popular hair-dye products. They may be further divided into three subcategories: permanent, demi-permanent, and auto-oxidative hair dyes. Permanent hair color contains ammonia and is mixed with developer, typically hydrogen peroxide, in various volumes in order to permanently change hair color. Depending upon the pH of the mixture and the strength of the developer, these systems have the capability to simultaneously lighten the hair's natural pigment and deposit color. The ammonia is an alkalizing agent that swells the hair fiber and opens the cuticle layer, allowing the color molecules and developer to penetrate into the cortex. Once inside, the developer lightens natural pigment and develops the color molecules so they remain permanently in the cortex. Permanent hair-color technologies' common uses include gray coverage, change of natural hair color, and lightening natural hair color. L'Oreal Excellence Crème hair color, Garnier Color Naturals Nourishing Permanent Hair Color Cream, Revlon ColorSilk, and Clairol Nice'n Easy are some examples of product in this category.

Demi-permanent formulas are ideal for enhancing, refreshing, or darkening hair color (either natural or previously colored). These formulas do not contain ammonia and use low-volume peroxide. Generally, they last up to six weeks, so they offer less commitment than permanent hair color. Because the developer is low strength, it is mild and the hair remains in optimal condition. Demi-permanents are also called "deposit-only permanent colors" as they do not lighten the hair, but only deposit color. Majority of the men's hair color in the market belongs to this class of dyes. Demi-permanent hair color is the fastest-growing color category in the industry because of its versatility. It is excellent for glazing or for refreshing previously tinted hair for added vibrancy and shine, and is essential for color correction. L'Oreal Healthy look crème gloss, Bigen Powder Hair Color, Just for Men Natural Hair Color, and Clairol Natural Instincts Hair Color are some examples of product in this category.

Auto-oxidative hair dyes involve the oxidation of dye precursors by oxygen in air without the use of an oxidant. This technology is based on precursors such as 1, 2, 4-trihydroxybenzene, 2,4-diaminophenol, 2-methoxy-p-phenylene diamine. Unlike, classic oxidative dyeing, hair is not lightened, so such systems are used to color gray hair or to change color from lighter to darker shades. Formulas containing these dyes involve no mixing, they are sold in one component and free of ammonia and hydrogen peroxide, and hence are milder than both demi-permanent and permanent hair-color products. Just for Men AutoStop hair color is an example of product in this category.

Concern over the safety of PPD and other hair-dye ingredients, the damage of hair due to oxidative coloring, and the demand for more convenient hair dyeing methods has fostered an increase in research in this area on new dyes and alternative hair-coloring technologies. Manufacturers have in recent decades embarked on intense research toward new dyes and precursors, as well as into alternative technologies for permanent hair dyeing. This research has been aimed not only at addressing potential toxicological issues but also technical weaknesses such as to mitigate hair damage, long-lasting color, no ammonia, no peroxide hair color, ease of application, and convenience.

6.15.3 FACTORS INFLUENCING COLOR FADING AND COLOR REMOVAL

Permanent hair-coloring products are formulated to provide excellent gray coverage, change existing hair color through removal of current hair color (lift) and deposit of new colors. Additionally, permanent hair-color products are formulated to give long-lasting and vibrant hair colors that provide overall youthful appearance. Several factors starting from formulation, product application, frequent washing, daily grooming habits, and environmental factors such as sun and pollution can accelerate color changes, color fading, vibrancy, and shine.

- **Color formulation and color application.**

When formulating hair-color products, several factors need to be taken into account in designing the appropriate vehicle. If color has not been given enough time to penetrate the hair shaft, color molecules will stay inside the cuticle layers and on the surface, allowing them to be washed away quickly. Most of fading appears after the first two washes, indicating that the color molecules settled on the outside of the hair shaft and had not penetrated deeply enough to be retained through washes. U.S. patent by Padmaja et al. teaches a two-step hair-color method, where the color precursors are applied in a first step that provides adequate time for effective penetration inside the hair fiber. In a second step, the hair is treated with hydrogen peroxide, so the reaction takes place inside the fiber and the dyes are trapped in the cortex, making them resistance to washing. The authors have shown more vibrant and longer-lasting color effect from this two-step system compared to conventional one-step hair coloring. In traditional permanent hair-coloring products as soon as the dye precursors are mixed with the developer, two competing factors come into play, the diffusion of dye precursors and peroxide into the fiber, the reaction of color precursor with peroxide outside the fiber. An optimal balance between the two factors contributes to overall color quality, long-lasting color, and color vibrancy.

- **Cuticle damage.**

The cuticle is the primary protection for the hair cortex where the majority of color molecules are housed. If friction or excessive chemical treatments damage the cuticle and strip away its protective fatty layer, the exposed cortex will chip away, and color molecules will escape during shampooing. Damaged hair is more porous and hydrophilic and hence absorbs more color during coloring and loses more color during washing. Protection of the cuticle with shampoos and conditioners that contain friction-reducing silicones helps reduce this type of color loss. Repair of hair damage using daily shampoos and conditioners containing protective polymers improves the state of the fiber and minimizes color loss due to the damage aspects of hair.

- **Rinsing with water.**

Fading due to water exposure is often related to a damaged cuticle. When the cuticle is overly compromised, water can more easily enter the cortex and some of the color molecules can be pulled out and washed away. Shampoos do not strip color. Studies show that water alone is responsible for the majority of color lost during shampooing.

- **Exposure to sunlight (UV and visible light).**

UV light is known to fade color in many substrates such as wood, cloth and paint. Hair is no different. UV radiation penetrates the hair and breaks down color molecules. The process happens with both natural and artificial pigments in the cortex and is the reason people develop highlights after spending long periods of time in the sun. UV protectants are added to some shampoos and styling products to help prevent hair color fade due to sunlight, although their efficacy is debated.

- **Some hair-color shades fade more quickly than others.**

Red shades tend to fade more than brown or black shades due to their relatively small molecule size, which can diffuse from the hair and wash away more quickly than other shades. UV exposure also breaks down the red tone more easily, while pure browns and blacks resist fading because their color molecules tend to be larger. Blonde shades have little color, so fading is less of a concern.

6.15.4 COLOR PROTECTION

Consumer demand for high-performance, vibrant, and fashion-oriented, yet natural-looking hair colorants continues to grow. To meet this trend, formulators must create high-impact products that provide lasting, natural-looking color as well as improved hair shine and conditioning effects. In recent years, the number of hair care products specifically designed to address such needs of color-treated hair is steadily increasing. The number of products claiming color protection continues to increase, and consumer product makers employ a variety of formulation strategies to address the needs of people who have color-treated hair. Rinse-off products such as shampoos and conditioners dominate the market and typically contain ingredients that emphasize the benefits of moisture retention, deposition of protective films on hair surface, and protection of color from sun fading using UV filters. Leave-on products, on the other hand, emphasize ingredients that serve to seal hair through deposition of polymers. Both formulation strategies address consumers who want to maintain the vitality of natural-looking hair following hair-color treatment. Naturally, consumers have a strong interest in adopting a hair care regimen that can extend the color vibrancy of hair, yet color fading and the loss of color vibrancy typically comes with everyday cleansing.

Studies by X et al. showed that color fading primarily occurs through physical removal of dyes by rinsing with water. These authors have investigated the physical and chemical factors that influence hair-color removal during the washing process by testing hair dye dissolution in water from dyed hair samples with variation of surfactant type, pH, and hair type. They have investigated a series of polymers with various functional groups and demonstrated that polymers with hydrophobically modified and cationic functionalities are the most effective in preventing hair-dye dissolution in water. A primary example of a polymer within this category is a cationic terpolymer of vinylpyrrolidone, dimethylaminopropyl methacrylamide, and methacryloylaminopropyl lauryldimonium chloride (INCI: Polyquaternium-55). Figure 1 shows the anti-fading test results of the four polymers in a leave-in treatment at 2% level using bleached hair tresses. The results demonstrate that Polyquaternium 55 (VP/DMAPA/C12-MAPTAC copolymer) leave-in treatment provides the highest color protection with 38% higher color improvement at the end of 10× washes over the control, and the effect is well perceivable by eye as shown in the picture.

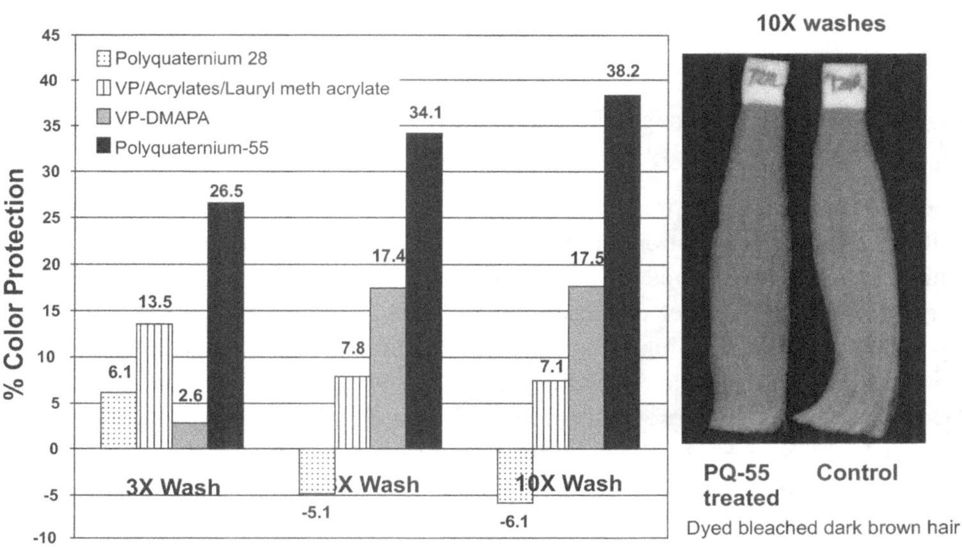

Figure 1. Pictures and percentages of color protection for dyed hair samples after 10× SLES washes and leave-in treatment of 2% of various polymers.

Both visual and instrumental measurement results indicate that Polyquaternium-55 provides a high level of color protection when formulated in a hair-color protection regimen with up to 50% color protection. Conditioning shampoos and conditioners with cationic surfactants and water proofing amino silicones can help combat the effects of water exposure.

Croda Inc. has commercialized a quaternized diester (ChromAveil) claimed to provide broad-spectrum sun protection to hair in rinse-off systems. It is a broad-spectrum UV filter that protected hair from color fading and hair integrity damage. Figure 2 below shows that hair treated with the diester shampoo protects the color from UV fading as evidenced by the lower value of Delta E, the total color change.

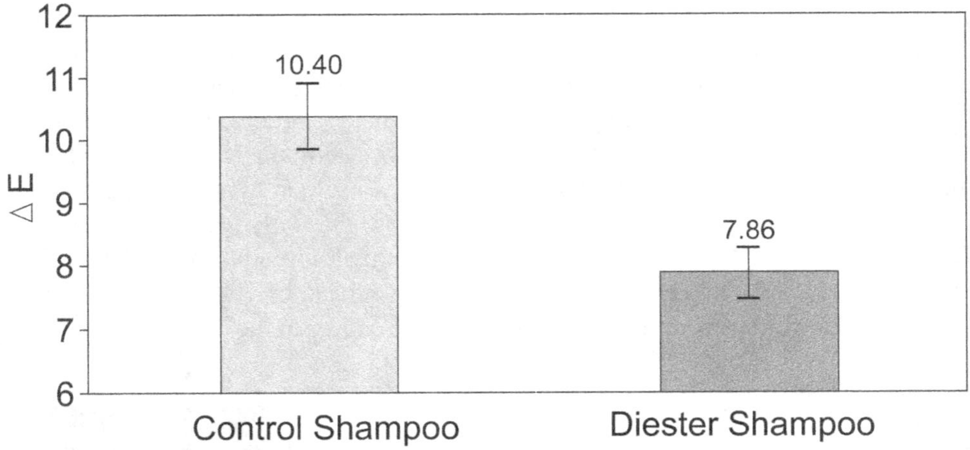

Figure 2. Total color change of medium brown-colored hair treated with different shampoos after 15 days of UV exposure

Silicones can help protect hair treated with permanent and nonpermanent colorants from discoloration and fading. Some color stays on the upper layers of cuticle and can be removed during washing. With its spreading behavior, silicone may help colorant further penetrate the hair cuticle for longer-lasting retention. By forming a water-insoluble film, the silicone may also help prevent color from washing out due to the hydrophobic nature of the silicone deposits on hair surface. Based on tests with several silicones, Figure 3 shows color retention properties for two silicones at 2% active level in a rinse-off conditioner. In this series of results, expressed by ΔE value, the silicones significantly reduced color loss compared to the control (the same rinse-off conditioner without silicone). The lower ΔE value for hair treated with the silicones indicates they help maintain color intensity and depth.

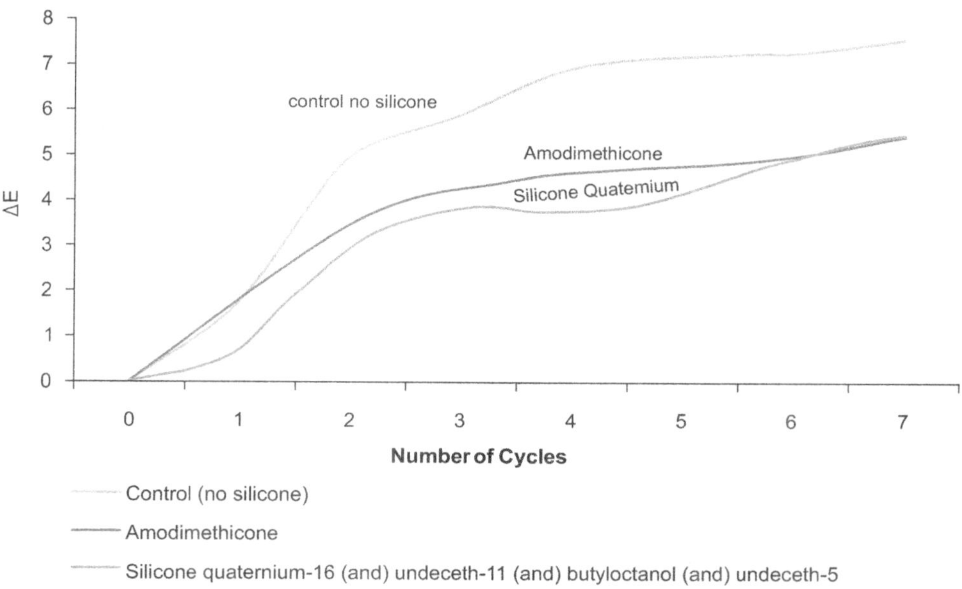

Figure 3. ΔE through seven cycles (each cycle = 7 hours of UV exposure + shampoo rinse + conditioner rinse at 2% active silicone)

A siloxane copolymer from Evonik grafted with methoxycinnamic acid ester and cationic alkoylamidopropyl dimethyl ammonium groups called Polysilicone-19 (trade name ABIL UV Quat 50) was investigated for color protection from UV. An active level (0.5–1%) of this silicone was incorporated in a shampoo and conditioner formulation. Colored hair tresses were treated with the shampoo and conditioner and irradiated by UV for a period of time. Color fading was compared to an untreated hair tress and other competitor ingredients. In a shampoo formulation at 0.5%, the silicone offered 50% reduced color fading and at 1.0% level from a conditioner application it offered 40% reduced color fading. The new silicone, Silicone Quaternium-22 microemulsion (trade name: ABIL® ME 45), offers significant color protection against washing. As a result, the combination of Silicone Quaternium-22 microemulsion and Polysilicone-19 in shampoos and conditioners can provide comprehensive color protection from UV and washing and premium hair-conditioning benefits with both visible and tangible benefits for consumers.

New color protection products include leave-on systems. Leave-on systems allow formulators to include functional ingredients like cationic film-forming polymers that bind with negatively charged amino acids on the surface of hair. These types of film-forming polymers can be found primarily in hair-styling gel and mousse formulations designed for hair hold, but they can also be used in personal care applications where a need exists to form a protective barrier on the hair cuticle. This protective barrier phenomenon can be strongly applied to products claiming hair-color protection. The film formed on the hair is believed to protect hair color from losing its vibrancy as a result of excess washing.

6.15.5 COLOR VIBRANCY AND SHINE

Human perception of color depends on the ability of our eyes and brains to detect and interpret the reflection of light on objects. When light shines on hair, part of it penetrates and is absorbed by the dye molecules, and part is reflected back. Shine-inducing shampoos and conditioners can be used on almost all hair types, creating the illusion of healthier hair. Darker hair tends to be shinier than lighter hair because it reflects light better, but as long as the cuticle and shaft are smooth, light is properly reflected off each individual strand. Hair shine is an important feature of hair appearance and this attractive visual effect is a key consumer objective in the hair care market. Hair-color intensity is another important attribute for colored hair.

Certain products and ingredients can enhance this effect. Conditioners are especially important when it comes to achieving shine because they replace natural oils and sebum that is lost further down the hair shaft. They penetrate, adding back lost moisture and giving the hair the ability to reflect light and therefore look shinier.

Consumers always want to have their colored hair appear bright and striking, or vibrant. Until now, neither a parameter nor a test method has been defined and developed to make such quantified "vibrancy" claims. Lefaudeus et al. have published principles for measuring hair luster (shine) using a Color Hair Visual Appearance Study System (SAMBA Hair system). SAMBA Hair System based on an innovative polarization camera SAMBA. They have observed that there are two bands on captured colored hair images: the "Shine" band (first reflection, no color) and the "Chroma" band (second reflection with color). The authors have defined an "Overlapping Coefficient" to describe overlapping degrees between "Shine" and "Chroma," the scalar product of the shine distribution and the chroma distribution. They have observed that the overlapping coefficient increases after specific cosmetic treatments and the treated hair demonstrated correspondingly shiner and richer color. Based on these observations and the established interaction mechanism between hair fiber and the light, a new parameter called "Hair Vibrancy Factor (HCVF)" is defined to describe shine and color intensity. Figure 4 shows the hair vibrancy factor measured on auburn-colored hair swatches after treatment with two hair-shine sprays using SAMBA.

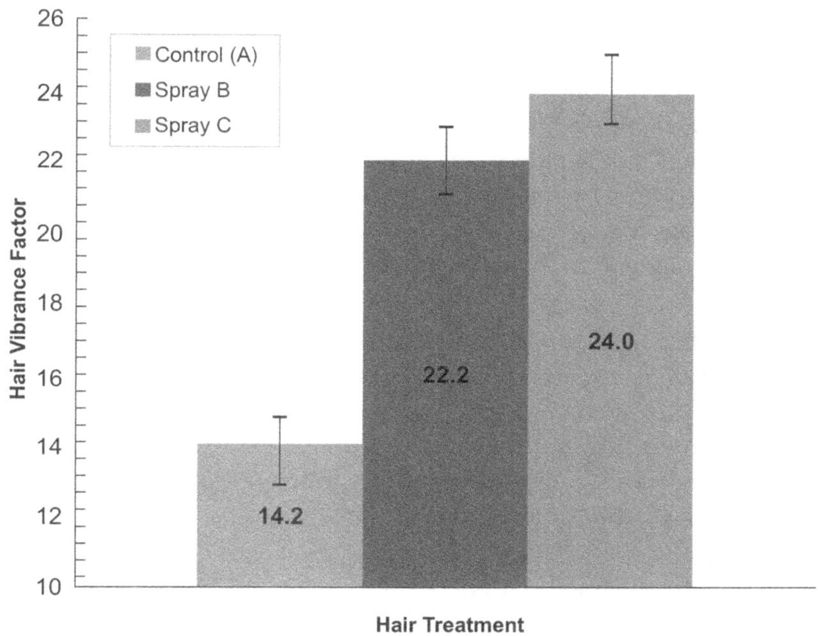

Figure 4. HCVF values of various hair samples measured using SAMBA

6.15.6 REMEDIES FOR COLOR PROTECTION, VIBRANCY, AND SHINE

The color-treated hair structure has a unique set of needs and characteristics. Dry hair that feels like straw and a dull, drab appearance are common complaints among those with color-treated hair. During oxidative hair coloring, the chemicals can also penetrate deep into color-treated hair and change the internal structure. Hair-strengthening proteins are attacked and porosity also increases, affecting hair's ability to hold the color molecules within the fiber. This leads to weaker hair that is more susceptible to hair-color fade. Red hair is especially susceptible to color fade, as the intense red pigments are the smallest and easily escape from a porous hair structure. Color-treated hair needs specialized care, so shampoos with gentle cleansing that protects the integrity of the color while still removing dirt, styling aids, and excess oils should be used. Damaged hair lacks moisture, so color-treated hair shampoos also infuse fresh hydration to help rejuvenate the hair's natural moisture. This grouping of products is further broken down into specialized formulas that provide additional capabilities, such as adding volume, protecting against UV damage, preserving color, enhancing color, augmenting highlights, and correcting tone.

Many color-safe shampoos and conditioners, particularly those that are geared toward a certain shade of hair color, will contain small bits of color and color enhancers to give your hair color a refreshed look after washing. They are wonderful for slowing the color-fading process. In addition to a good, color-safe shampoo and conditioner, you should select supporting daily products that contain sunscreens and light oils. Keep your hair thoroughly moisturized using conditioners that are specifically designed to address the needs of color-treated hair. Regular conditioning goes a long way toward preserving hair color and keeping the hair radiant.

Finally, use finishing products like hairsprays, spritzes, mousses, and gels sparingly. The alcohols used in these style-setting products are used to help your hair dry faster in your style, but can fade your hair color prematurely. Some have also reported that volumizing product lines, or those for fine hair, also fade new hair colors quickly because they allow a slight lifting of the cuticle layers to provide the illusion of increased hair-shaft thickness.

6.15.7 INGREDIENTS AND PRODUCTS FOR COLOR-TREATED HAIR

Ingredients for color protection, shine, and vibrancy include the well-established ones such as: silicones for color protection and shine, quaternary ammonium compounds for ease of combing, and conditioning and vegetable oils for shine. Formulating shampoos and conditioners with just 2% of Dow Corning's CE-8411 nonionic silicone emulsion provide color protection benefits, enhance hair shine, and help prevent hair breakage. Many ingredients are recently launched to address hair and scalp aging at the cellular level, improve follicle health, reduce hair loss, and offer antioxidant properties.

Natural vegetable oils provide nourishing conditioning and shine to hair. Coconut oil, being a triglyceride of lauric acid (principal fatty acid), has a high affinity for hair proteins and, because of its low molecular weight and straight linear chain, is able to penetrate inside the hair shaft.[21] Avocado and Jojoba oil are other oils for nourishing, conditioning, and shine benefits. Sunscreens are another category of ingredients now found in a variety of hair care products, including shampoos, conditioners, and hairsprays. They prevent breakdown of keratin due to sun exposure and also keep hair dye from fading in ultraviolet light. Ingredients like Crodasorb™ UV-HPP from Croda and PARSOL® SLX provide multiple benefits like prevention of color fading, strengthening hair, and enhancing gloss when delivered through hair color, or hair care products, especially leave-on sprays. Table 1 below lists some advanced functional hair care ingredients for color protection and shine popular in today's hair care market.

Table 1. Advanced hair care ingredients used for color protection and shine

Hair Care Ingredients	**Benefits**	**Supplier**
ABIL® UV Quat 50	Efficient protection of hair color against fading in sun light. Protection of fiber integrity against damage by V irradiation.	Evonik
Linseed Oil™	Linseed Oil provides hair-color protection and radiant shine to color-treated hair.	Textron
ChromAveil ®	Protects the hair from the damaging effects of sunlight. Gives color protection benefits to dyed hair from UVA and protects the mechanical properties of the hair from UVB.	Croda Inc.
Crodasorb™ UV-HPP	Polyester polyquaternized ingredient that is substantive to hair and protects against the damaging effects of UV-B radiation	Croda Inc.
Lustreplex®	Creates lustrous, healthy looking hair from anionic systems. Provides frizz control, shine, detangling, and conditioning benefits.	Croda Inc.
Dow Corning® CE-8411 Smooth Plus Emulsion	Repair colored, gray, and heat-damaged hair by restoring moisturized feel, shine, & alignment. Protects hair from further damage and color loss.	Dow Corning
Dow Corning® 5-7113 Silicone Quat Microemulsion	Restore smoothness, shine and Alignment. Prolong hair color. Protects hair from breakage.	Dow Corning
Coconut Oil	Provides conditioning, smoothness, and vibrant shine to color-treated hair.	Natural Sourcing
PARSOL® SLX	PARSOL® SLX is a silicone-based UV-B absorber delivers multiple benefits including prevention of color fading, gloss enhancement, and conditioning.	DSM

The hair care market is overloaded with products specifically designed to care for color-treated hair and protect the color from fading, so color can last longer. Redken has launched Color Extend, a collection of four products—shampoo, conditioner, treatment, and color protection—for complete care of color-treated hair. Shampoo for color-treated hair protects hair color from fading and provides UVA/UVB ray protection. Conditioner resurfaces the cuticle for a smooth, vibrant finish and helps with color retention; anti-fade protection maximizes color vibrancy and strengthens hair.

Protective treatment provides deep conditioning to leave hair manageable and vibrant. Specially formulated to provide stronger protection to extend life of hair color, this treatment for color-treated hair uses Fade Resist Complex with UVA & UVB filters to help lock in color and block out aggressors. Hair-color protection spray delivers anti-fade color protection and cuticle reinforcement to maintain color vibrancy and shine.

Pantene has recently launched a range of seven products for color-treated hair, Smooth Shampoo & Conditioner, Volume Shampoo & Conditioner, Color Seal Concentrate, two-minute Damage Rescue Treatment, and Instant Nourishing Shine Spray. The active formula in this shampoo helps to preserve the color for long-lasting brilliance. The active formula in this shampoo helps to preserve the color for long-lasting brilliance. This hair-moisturizing shampoo cleanses your hair while also infusing it with hydration. It features special moisturizers that build a layer around the hair fibers to protect hair from damage and color loss. Shampooing with the Pantene shampoo will add vibrancy and volume to color-treated hair.

6.15.8 CONCLUSIONS

Consumer demand for high-performance, vibrant and fashion-oriented, yet natural-looking hair colorants continues to grow. The global increase in hair-color products raises the need for color care products in the market. The number of hair care products specifically designed to address such needs of color-treated hair is steadily increasing and products claiming long-lasting color, shine, and color enhancement continue to increase. Rinse-off products such as shampoos and conditioners dominate the market and typically contain ingredients that emphasize the benefits of moisture retention, deposition of protective films on hair surface, and protection of color from sun fading using UV filters. Leave-on products, on the other hand, emphasize ingredients that serve to seal hair through deposition of polymers. Both formulation strategies address consumers who want to maintain the vitality of natural-looking hair following hair color. Despite the improvements made on color protection using specialized hair care products containing silicones, vegetable oils, and cationic polymers, a complete color protection is still far from reality. This is due to the fact that color loss, and loss in shine and vibrancy, are linked to hair damage and the majority of hair-color products in the market induce hair damage during the hair-coloring process. Over the years, hair-color product manufacturers have continually improved hair-color formulations to minimize hair damage. A complete damage-free hair color remains as a dream despite of the technological advancements. Regular use of color-treated hair care products significantly improves the appearance of color-treated hair, providing shine and vibrancy, and it prolongs the life color by 40–50%. This chapter provides an overview of the fundamentals of hair coloring, the factors influencing hair fading, and finally a compilation of some hair ingredients and color-protection products currently available in the market.

REFERENCES

Abil Quat. H.I. Leidreiter, U.Kortemeier, U.Maczkiewitz, M.Pascaly, Protection of Hair Fiber Appearance and Strength against UV-Damage, Proc of 23rd. IFSCC Congress (2004).

S. Herrwerth, I. Ulrich-Brehm, U. Kortemeier, P. Winter, M. Ferenz, B. Grüning, Silicone Quaternium-22: New Silicone Technology for Premium Hair Conditioning with Additional Benefits, SOFW J, 2009, 6, 11–18.

PART 6.16

REACTIVE HAIR PRODUCTS

Author
Charles Warren

TABLE OF CONTENTS

Reactive hair care products are those products that chemically react with or in the hair to provide a desired effect. These products are hair colors, bleaches, relaxers/straighteners, and permanent waves.

6.16.1 COLORS

Temporary Hair Colors

There are generally two types of products in this category: hair cosmetics and temporary stains.

Hair cosmetics are generally suspensions of colored pigments (e.g., iron oxides) and/or tinted glitter particles in an aqueous or hydroalcoholic solution containing holding resins (e.g., VP/VA copolymer). These formulas are applied directly to the hair and upon drying provide visual effects—"color" or "sparkle," depending on the formulation. The pigments/glitter are actually incorporated in the film on the hair and, therefore, can be easily removed by breaking the film and brushing the particulate out or by simply washing the hair to remove the film and the particulate.

"6 Wash" Colors

Temporary stains are actually mixtures of direct colors (i.e., the color molecules are the color they will remain) applied to the hair to stain the exterior (cuticle) with minimal penetration to the cortex. These "direct dyes" are usually applied in a shampoo or shampoo-like solution and can be simply washed in (color-enhancing shampoos) or applied and left on the hair for a period of time to achieve the depth and color desired. Color-enhancing shampoos provide minimal "gray" coverage and are used primarily to refresh existing color. Temporary colors (referred to as "6 Wash Colors") provide coverage to gray that is less than 10% of the whole hair volume and will remain on the hair for approximately six washes. Each washing or wetting of the hair will remove some of the stain, so care must be taken that the dyes are removed in a similar fashion so that the color remains as true as possible.

"Demi"-Permanent (non-ammoniacal, 12 wash colors)

Demi-permanent hair colors are two component colors. The first component, the color solution, is an aqueous mixtures of traditional hair-dye intermediates (e.g., paraphenylenediamine or PPD), monethanolamine (MEA), surfactants, and additives. The mixture of the dye intermediates is critical to the development of the desired colors and is very similar to the standard permanent hair-color mixtures. The MEA makes the solution slightly alkaline to assist with the color development when mixed with the developer.

The second component, the developer, is an aqueous solution of hydrogen peroxide (generally, 3–6%).

When mixed together, the MEA helps make the hydrogen peroxide more reactive with the dye intermediates to develop the highly colored polymerized color molecules that ultimately are the desired color. The MEA also serves to swell the hair and allow permeation of the developing color polymers into the subcuticular layers of the hair. Because the hydrogen peroxide is at a relatively low concentration and the MEA only slightly raises the pH (7–8), this coloring process results in little, if any, bleaching of the native hair color—thus, the "tone-on-tone" nomenclature for these type colors. Demi-permanent colors will not allow for a shade lighter than the starting shade. Demi-permanent colors will last for 12–20 shampoos and will provide coverage of gray hair that is less than 25–30% of the total hair volume.

Because demi-permanent hair colors function at lower pH and lower peroxide levels, there is relatively little damage to the hair. This category of hair color has seen the largest share of growth in the consumer market over the past 20 years.

Permanent Colors

Similar to the demi-permanent colors, the permanent color products are two component systems: the color solution and the developer solution.

The color solution is an aqueous mixture of reactive dye intermediates (e.g., PPD), ammonia, and additives. As in the demi-permanent colors, it is the mixture (quantities and types of intermediates) that yields the ultimate final color. The pH of this color solution is usually around 9, one of the significant differences between demi- and permanent colors.

The developer solution is an aqueous solution of hydrogen peroxide. The peroxide content of the developer solution can vary from 6% to 12%. There are some higher peroxide level developers, but those are predominantly only in the professional salon market and relatively few in number. Peroxides are also referred to by "volume" of oxygen delivered. For practical purposes, 6% = 20 volume, 9% = 30 volume, and 12% = 40 volume. In the retail market, 6% is the most common peroxide level.

When the two components are combined, the peroxide becomes extremely reactive and quickly initiates polymerization of the dye intermediates and, simultaneously, the bleaching of the native color. The high pH of the mixture swells the hair and allows the dye intermediates and peroxide to quickly penetrate throughout the hair shaft. The highly colored, polymerized dyes become too large to leave the hair and therefore replace the color of the hair. The higher the level of peroxide used will dictate the degree of bleaching that will be accomplished. Permanent hair coloring can lighten the hair significantly and can result in significant color change. These colors are durable and will usually last six weeks or through 24–30 wash cycles. By this time in the process, root growth has become the factor that usually requires the re-colorization process.

Permanent hair coloring is the most damaging of all of the additive coloring processes. This damage can be ameliorated by using a "conditioning" base, or a special conditioning treatment for post-coloring application.

6.16.2 BLEACHES

Bleaching is the process by which the native melanin in the hair is partially or completely destroyed, leaving the hair slightly to radically lighter than the starting point. Highlighting is the bleaching of selected portions of the hair to create a mixture of light and darker hair throughout the entire coiffure. Multiple techniques of application are used to create multiple effects, but the fundamental destruction of native melanin remains the same.

Bleaching can be accomplished by mixing an aqueous, ammonia (ph = 9–10), surfactant solution with 6%–12% hydrogen peroxide and monitoring the color removal until the desired shade is attained. Bleach powders, blends of highly reactive peroxydisulfates (sodium, potassium, and ammonium salts), can be mixed with peroxide to provide faster and more complete melanin destruction. Bleach oils, mixtures of lipoidal materials, and surfactants can also be employed to provide easier spreading throughout the hair and easier removal once the desired shade is attained.

Due to the high pH and high levels of peroxide (which not only destroys melanin, but can oxidize the inherent protein comprising hair), bleaching is one of the most damaging processes done on the hair. The hair is left in a weaker state and is therefore subject to more dryness and breakage than before the bleaching operation. Overbleaching, resulting from too high a level of bleaching or repeated bleach processing to the same hair, can and will result in breakage.

6.16.3 STRAIGHTENERS

Hair straightening has existed since the time of the ancient Egyptians. Extremely kinky, curly hair (e.g., Afro-Caribbean hair) or highly curly hair (e.g., European hair) can be very difficult to manage and style. Straighteners have been developed to release the natural curl of the hair and leave it more amenable to traditional styling.

Relaxers

The use of alkaline material to straighten curly/kinky hair has been documented from the time of the ancient Egyptian dynasties when women at court applied mud mixed with ash to the hair and left in place until the desired straightness was achieved. Today's relaxers are technically superior, but apply the same basic chemical principles.

The backbone of all human hair, the reason that hair has its configuration, tensile strength, elasticity, etc. is attributed primarily to the cystine (-S-S-) cross-linked bonds throughout the hair. Clearly to change the configuration of the hair, these bonds need to be altered. Highly alkaline conditions can convert the cystine linkages (-S-S-) to lanthionine linkages (-S-) while the hair is being mechanically placed into a new configuration.

As indicated, relaxing hair is both a chemical and mechanical process. The cystine bonds must be broken (chemical) and the hair must be placed and held in a new configuration (mechanical) until the new lanthionine bonds (chemical) are reformed, keeping the hair in its new configuration.

Sodium hydroxide (also known as lye) is one of the oldest alkaline agents used to straighten hair. At a concentration between 1.8% and 2.1%, sodium hydroxide–containing relaxers can effectively straighten hair to a level of manageability 15–20 minutes. The earliest versions of relaxers were simply lye (NaOH) mixed in with a thick animal fat (e.g., lard). Subsequent versions became more sophisticated, but still required a step called "basing," wherein a layer of non-lye-containing grease was placed as a protective barrier on the scalp and on the skin around the hairline. Modern relaxers do not require this "basing" step and are therefore referred to as "No-Base" relaxers.

The modern alkali relaxer is a mixture of an aqueous phase containing the alkali ingredient (sodium hydroxide, potassium hydroxide, or lithium hydroxide), propylene glycol, and other water-soluble ingredients and an oil-phase-containing petrolatum, mineral oil, and fatty alcohols held together in a slightly stable emulsion by an emulsifier. The oil phase is mixed and then the aqueous phase is added. The mixture is mixed hot until semi-emulsified and then cooled. As it cools the non-emulsified petrolatum thickens along with the emulsion and serves to physically hold the entire mixture together. The resultant mixture can best be described as a dual emulsion (part oil-in-water and part water-in-oil). This quasi-emulsion is by design so that when applied and worked through the hair, both oil and water containing the alkali will be released onto the hair to accomplish the chemical breakage of the cystine bonds. The thickness of the petrolatum helps hold the hair straight while the lanthionization process is completed and hair is chemically held in a new straighter configuration. When the desired straightness is attained the mixture is rinsed out and washed out with an acidic shampoo to neutralize any remaining alkali.

Alkali relaxation is damaging to the hair and is corrosive to skin if allowed to remain in contact for too long a period. Overrelaxation can result in immediate hair breakage or significant hair breakage over a short period after the process. Skin damage can result in mild edema or significant burning if contact time is prolonged. Once successfully completed, the hair requires conditioning and addition of significant levels of oil to remain soft, pliable, and have a pleasing appearance. Regrowth will still be kinky/curly and is usually the driving force for a new application (new growth only) in four to six weeks.

In the 1970s the modern consumer "no lye" relaxer was developed. These relaxers are two component relaxers. The relaxer crème is simply the oil phase (quasi-emulsified), similar to the alkali relaxer in which is suspended relatively insoluble calcium hydroxide particles. The activator is an aqueous solution of guanidine carbonate. When the two components are mixed immediately before application, guanidine hydroxide is formed, which chemically performs exactly like the alkali relaxers, creating the new lanthionine linkage in the new configuration. This process is slower than a straight alkali relaxer, as it takes time for the guanidine hydroxide to form and react with the cystine in the hair. This lower reactivity makes the relaxer less potentially damaging to the hair and scalp and is the main reason that most relaxers sold at the retail, use-at-home level are of this type. However, the potential safety issues are still there and hair breakage and skin damage are still possible. The opportunity to prevent these negative occurrences is greater with this type of relaxer. Thorough rinsing and shampoo with an acidic shampoo is still required. Guanidine hydroxide is unstable and will decompose in a matter of hours, so the mixed relaxer must be used immediately and disposed when process is complete.

Relaxers based on conventional reducing agents (thioglycolates and bisulfites) have been marketed. These relaxers are based on the reduction of the cystine bonds by the reducing substance, mechanical reconfiguration of hair, and subsequent reformation of the cystine bonds by the use of hydrogen peroxide (with thioglycolate) or alkaline shampoo (with bisulfate). The reducing agent is generally in an aqueous gel form, applied to the hair, combed straight and then placed under moderate heat. The reducing solution is then rinsed and followed with the neutralization step, an aqueous solution of hydrogen peroxide 2–3% or an alkaline shampoo (pH 8). These reducing relaxers are not as effective on kinky, curly hair and moderately effective on curly wavy hair.

The "Japanese" straightening system employs a reducing solution followed immediately by pressing the hair in a hot flat iron in thin sections. Peroxide neutralization follows. This system is highly effective but requires significant time and operator expertise.

The most recent relaxer/straightening system is the "Brazilian" or "Keratin" straightening system. This system is an aqueous solution of hydrolyzed keratin and a significant quantity of formaldehyde or formaldehyde precursor chemicals. When heat is applied via hot flat iron, the resultant formaldehyde cross-links the protein and holds it in the new, straighter configuration. While highly effective in straightening and retaining hair in straight configuration, formaldehyde has significant safety issues, especially in the gaseous form, created when the hot flat irons are used.

Blow Dry Lotions

Straightening lotions, creams, gels used with blow dryers are generally mixtures of high-molecular-weight silicones that allow the hair to be continually brushed while heat is applied via a blow dryer. This approach will straighten moderately curly hair, but the effect is temporary and highly susceptible to reversion of the hydrogen bonds from applied water or environmental humidity.

PART 6.17

FORMULA/PRODUCT DEVELOPMENT FROM THE FORMULATOR'S VIEWPOINT

(Expectations, Initial Prototypes, Final Prototypes)

Author
Charles Warren

ABSTRACT

Formulators must always be aware of what the consumer requires and expects from the formula being developed. Each category and subcategory has its own particular set of expectations and requirements. The best way to understand these is to listen and observe consumers talking about the particular products/formulas and to observe those same consumers as they talk about them. Marketing groups usually conduct focus groups where consumers will talk about their issues or their experiences with products. These discussions can be invaluable to a formulator who wants to create a successful product.

TABLE OF CONTENTS

6.17.1 FUNCTIONALITY/PERFORMANCE

Every product must deliver against its primary function—shampoos must clean, conditioners must provide a conditioning benefit, hand and body lotions must leave the skin moisturized, etc. Unfortunately, not every consumer will love every product because no two consumers are exactly alike. Formulators will develop functional products that will meet the performance requirements of a large number of consumers—that's the best they can hope for.

Form

Consumers will always gravitate to products that deliver on their promises. They are more likely to work with a product that is in a form that they are familiar with and is easy to use. The formulator must consider all of the aspects of consumer use while developing a particular formula. A cream or a lotion that is difficult to dispense or leaves a large amount of product unused in a package will quickly be abandoned by the consumer, and that consumer will look to one of the other hundreds of similar products available.

A good formulator will survey the competitive product arena in the specific area where they are formulating to determine what consumers are interested in and how those products are used and received. New and novel approaches are always of interest, but need to be evaluated thoroughly to ensure that the new form will be accepted by the desired number and category of consumers.

Beliefs

Learning, working with, and formulating against consumer beliefs can be a challenge for the formulator. These beliefs vary in individual markets and can vary wildly across cultural barriers. For example, in the United States most consumers believe that a shampoo or bodywash should deliver copious amounts of foam to deliver the cleaning they require. In other countries or cultures, excessive foam is viewed as a distinct negative. The formulator needs to be aware of the beliefs surrounding the formulating area of interest. Again, a survey of the successful products in a given market can provide insight into what the consumers may believe about the category.

A product that is sold as a moisturizing or conditioning will probably have to have a creamy texture and be opaque or translucent to have the consumer believe that it will actually perform. A clear conditioner or moisturizing lotion may provide excellent conditioning and moisturization, but would have a fairly high belief hurdle to conquer with the consumer. Clear products can be easily believed to deliver good cleaning properties, and expectations of conditioning or moisturization are low from the onset.

In addition to visual beliefs, are the olfactive beliefs. In some cultures lemon-scented cleanser will be thought of as cleaning while a vanilla-scented cleanser will be thought of as conditioning/moisturizing. A formulator must be careful to not unconsciously set up belief contradictions in the consumer's mind. Fragrance suppliers can be of great assistance in understanding the role that fragrance plays in the perception of product performance.

Post-usage beliefs are another issue for the formulator. If the hair or skin is left with a perceived coating or residue after usage, the consumer can believe that the hair or skin is coated and not aesthetically acceptable even though the residue may play an important role in delivering the functional benefit. Hairsprays or styling products that do not create a stiff film (e.g., "crust") will be perceived as not holding strongly enough even though consumers may say that they dislike the "crust" and would prefer products that do not impart that degree of stiffness.

Listening to the consumer, observing the consumer, and reading consumer comments are the best way to understand beliefs and find a way to use those beliefs to create more acceptable formulas.

6.17.2 MARKETING REQUIREMENTS/EXPECTATIONS

The Marketing groups, with whom formulators work, also have a large and varied set of requirements and expectations. In order for a formulator to develop formulas that address these, there must be constant communication and clarification with their Marketing partners in order to avoid unpleasant reactions or surprises related to the formula developed.

Functionality/Performance

Marketing will always expect the formula to deliver against the basic premise of the product—a fair expectation. They will always hope that the formula will perform better than the competition, support all of the claims that they would desire to make, and be less expensive to allow for lower price points and higher profits—more complicated expectations.

Communication between the formulator and the Marketing group early on and continuously throughout the development and finalization process can help manage expectations and can often lead to better formulas that fulfill most of the requirements (technical and marketplace) of the product. Upfront definition of product requirements, competitive performance requirements, advertising claims performance, and cost requirements are of utmost importance. If the organization does not have a "Product Description" process, a formulator will need to create one that provides information and standards that must be considered and used while formulation is in process.

Form/Package

Differentiation between products in the market is always desired. A new product form or a revolutionary new package are methods of differentiation in a crowded marketplace that can make a formula/product stand out. However, these forms and packages can create significant issues in development, testing, usage, and stability for the formulator. Part of the early definition of the product needs to identify all of the issues for a new form or package and, then, throughout the development process all of these issues (plus new ones discovered) must be communicated and resolved for both the formulator and the Marketing group.

Cost

Formula cost and total product cost (formula, packaging—primary and secondary, manufacturing, etc.) are a significant issue for the formulator. Again, early identification of formula cost allowable will dictate what the formulator can choose from the formulation toolbox. Rarely is total cost freedom provided to a formulator, so an eye must always be kept on the cost/benefit equation during the development of formulas.

Formula costs are generally thought of as the cost of the raw materials used to assemble the formula, and those costs are usually what appear in the financial analysis of a new product. However, other costs need to be identified early on to keep the entire process cost-effective. Testing costs (consumer use testing, claims testing, specialized analytical testing, competitive products, required efficacy testing, safety testing, packaging for testing, etc.) can all be hidden costs that need to be identified, discussed, and approved prior to and during formula development.

Stability/Shelf-Life

Expectations that a formula and entire product will remain stable and consumer acceptable throughout the shelf-life of a product are reasonable and required. A formulator must create formulas that will remain stable (i.e., not separate, not change color, not develop malodor, not negatively interact with packaging, continue to dispense and perform properly, etc.) from manufacture through warehousing through shipping, through shelf storage to consumer purchase and usage. In the case of OTC drugs, this is beyond an expectation; it is a legal requirement. The formulator needs to be aware of these requirements and test the formula (as reasonably as possible) to ensure that appropriate stability has been attained.

There are many references available for the formulator to review regarding stability and shelf-life testing. Most organizations have their own requirements and protocols for stability testing and, in the case of OTC drugs, there are specific stability-testing requirements.

Claims

Advertising claims (on package, in print, in media) are another important way of differentiating products in the same category. The fundamental regulation related to claims for a product is that there must be support for every product claim. The type, quantity and quality of the support is usually only defined when there is a challenge to a particular claim and that usually occurs after the fact. Some claims can be supported simply by product category—a bodywash formula containing surfactants will support general cleaning claims. Other "contains" claims (e.g., "with jojoba oil") can be supported by simply incorporating the claimed ingredient(s) in the formula. Performance claims or competitive claims are usually more difficult to support, but support must be developed nonetheless.

Desired claims are another area that must be discussed early on in the formulation process and the verbiage and method of support should be reviewed and agreed to among the formulating, marketing, regulatory and legal groups. Often times, the discussions around claims and support become discussions of risk and consequences.

Claims regarding product performance can be challenged in multiple ways. Legal departments from one company can challenge another company's claims via a simple letter, using the National Advertising Division (NAD) of the Better Business Bureau's self-regulating challenge process or by legal action. The NAD can challenge claims independently. Various countries and advertising regulating agencies have their own procedures for requiring claim support for claims used in advertising. Formulators can learn a great deal about support principles and claim support by reading the findings from these challenges.

6.17.3 MANUFACTURING REQUIREMENTS/EXPECTATIONS

Materials

The Manufacturing or Supply Chain groups within an organization reasonably require/expect that the materials selected for a formula are readily available and in quantity sufficient to support manufacturing of the formula. When a formula selects new or novel materials or works with a new, unfamiliar supplier, communication with the various Supply Chain groups will be necessary to ensure that the formula can be successfully manufactured on a continual basis without significant issues.

Equipment

The Supply Chain organizations will determine if a formula can be manufactured internally, using existing equipment, internally with new equipment, or externally at a contract manufacturer that has the appropriate equipment or registrations (e.g.,

OTC drug manufacture registration). The formulator will need to work with all of these groups to ensure proper and smooth manufacturing of their formulas.

Warehousing/Shipping

The final product (formula and packaging) will undoubtedly need to be stored at some point between manufacture and consumer purchase. The Supply Chain organization will expect that the formula will be stable throughout the storage under conditions that are normally experienced during this storage (i.e., unheated or non-cooled warehouse).

Regulatory/Legal Requirements

Throughout prior sections, the role of the Regulatory and Legal groups has been referenced. These groups are responsible for the compliance of the organization in all aspects related to the formula and the ultimate finished product. Formulators should engage these groups early on in the formulating process to ensure that everything possible is done to keep the product on track and compliant with any and all regulations.

OTC vs. Non-OTC

As indicated previously, cosmetic formulas and OTC formulas exist in close proximity. Formulators should be aware of those products that automatically fall under the governance of the OTC monographs and all of the formula requirements (e.g., active ingredients) that those monographs indicate. Consultation with Regulatory and Legal groups is imperative when operating in or close to this arena.

Safety

The manufacturer/distributor of a product is responsible for assuring the safety of the products it markets. The formulator is responsible for developing and testing formulas that support this responsibility. Most organizations have protocols that dictate the degree of safety evaluation and/or testing that is required for each formula prior to consumer exposure, either in testing or in actual product marketing. Communication with the groups within the organization responsible for product safety is essential for the formulator.

Intellectual Property

Intellectual property protection (e.g., patents) is essential to ensure an organization's rights to formulas/products developed by that company. The formulator has two responsibilities related to this protection: 1) to ensure that formulas developed do not infringe on the intellectual properties of individuals or organizations; and

2) to ensure that proprietary development can be and is protected for the formulas developed.

The first responsibility can be exercised by obtaining a Freedom to Practice approval from the appropriate body within the organization or via a consultant skilled in this determination. This will involve patent searches (domestic and foreign) conducted by skilled groups in consultation and discussion with the formulator.

The second responsibility is exercised by maintaining adequate and thorough documentation of the formulation from the earliest point in the process and continuing throughout the development and testing. Most organizations have processes for submitting and processing ideas that may or may not ultimately result in patents, and the prudent formulator will become familiar with these processes early on in the development process.

Initial Prototypes

Once the formulator has direction on the type, form, etc. of the formula to be developed, the actual formulation work and development of initial prototypes can be initiated.

The best places to start when developing initial prototypes within a given category are:

- Existing formulas in the organization's current or historical formulae portfolio
- Supplier formularies (available from supplier representative or through the supplier website) from suppliers supplying materials to the specific category (e.g., surfactant suppliers for shampoos, bodywashes, cleansers)

These formulas can be modified with additional materials to increase various aspects or used to identify materials and ratios of materials to use in new prototype development. The formulator can also look at competitive formulas in the category of interest to determine what materials are currently being used to achieve desired benefits.

Existing Bases/Forms

Existing organizations usually have or have had a portfolio of formulas in the categories of interest. Often a formulator can use one of these existing formulas as a starting point in the development of a new formula. The positives of this approach are related to the entire organizational familiarity with the materials, manufacturing, safety, etc. of the formula. The negatives are that the formula will probably not exhibit the novelty that will differentiate it from the products in the marketplace. These negatives can be assuaged by slight changes (e.g., fragrance, claims ingredients) to the formulas or new and novel claims that can be developed for the existing base formula.

Stocked/Currently Used Raw Materials

A formulator should start the formulation process by looking at the raw materials currently used by the organization. There is no need to source a new version of a material that is essentially identical to a material already sourced and used. Most organizations have many examples of multiple versions of the same raw material, differing only in source of supply. Differences in raw materials that make significant formulation differences are the cause for selecting one raw material over another even if they would apparently have little difference. The responsible formulator will identify these issues and make sure that the differences actually require the selection of new or different sources.

6.17.4 NEW RAW MATERIALS, BASES, FORMS

Raw Material Availability (quantity and geography)

Once a formulator has selected a new or novel raw material to use in a formula, the availability of the material in quantity sufficient to support manufacturing requirements in all of the markets where manufacturing will occur should be determined. Transporting materials internationally can impact the timing and ability for organizations to provide product to the marketplaces desired. The formulator can work with the supplier of the raw materials and the appropriate supply chain groups to ensure that all parties are comfortable with the ability to support the marketing of the formula.

Storage Requirements

Specialized storage requirements (e.g., refrigeration) for new raw materials or final formulas will need to be communicated to the organization early on in the development process.

Cost vs. Performance

New raw materials, bases, or forms are generally more expensive than existing versions. The formulator needs to evaluate the benefits (performance, manufacturability, claims, safety, etc.) versus the cost. This evaluation process is often ignored or conducted too late in the development process to be of value.

Regulatory Requirements/Issues

Using a new raw material, base, or form can result in an entirely new set of regulatory requirements (e.g., VOC maximums). Early on in the development process, a formulator should review these issues with the appropriate regulatory groups and then keep those groups advised throughout the developmental process.

Ease of Use in Manufacturing

New raw materials or formula bases can often create problems for the manufacturing groups. These problems can result from the material/base/form itself or, in the case of the raw material, how it is packaged or delivered (i.e., pails, drums, or bulk containers). All of these problems need to be discussed with the manufacturing groups early on to ensure the smooth transition from initial prototypes to production.

Claims Ingredients

Different ingredients can deliver different claims for a product, which can actually be important to performance or which simply allow advertisable claims. The formulator needs to know the differences and select the best way of proceeding.

Delivering Perceivable, Differentiated Claims in Formula

Raw materials in this category are the "gold standard" of claims ingredients. If the material can deliver a consumer-perceivable difference that can be measured (technically or through consumer testing) and used to support meaningful claims, the formulator has a significant win. This win will allow differentiation in the marketplace and consumer satisfaction versus the advertised claims.

Delivering Technical Claims in Formula

Raw materials in this category are important, as they allow product differentiation via technical claim support. The formula base itself may deliver the consumer-acceptable performance required and the inclusion of the technical support directly attributable to an ingredient will be of great value.

"Contains"

Raw materials in this category are the most ubiquitous in the marketplace. The materials may or may not deliver any benefit at the level used in the formula, but they are included for label or advertising purposes. Trendy new extracts, oils, etc. are widely used in products simply so that the "with X" claim can appear on the label or in advertising.

"Contains" ingredients and claims should require certain levels of use in the formula, depending on the placement on product. If the "claim" ingredient is an integral part of the product name, it should be used at a more significant level than if it is only included as a "with" claim. Any performance claims made for the use of these raw materials must be carefully evaluated to ensure that there are no false or misleading claims that could be subject to challenge or litigation.

6.17.5 FINAL PACKAGING

Material of Construction

Starting with initial prototypes, the formulator needs to be aware of the composition of the final package into which the formula will be placed. Transparent versus translucent versus opaque packaging could have significant impact on the stability of a formula. Determining what testing should be done during the early phases of prototype development is important for the formulator as the development process is initiated.

Dispensing Mechanism

Of equal importance is the means by which the formula is dispensed for use by the consumer. The formula needs to be easily and completely dispensed from the primary package. A thick cream may not be able to be pumped; a thin solution might not be appropriate for a wide mouth; etc. Once prototype formulas are developed, dispensing tests should be conducted with dispensing devices similar to those for the final products to make sure that there are no issues.

Special Manufacturing Considerations

The formulator needs to be aware of where the formula will ultimately be manufactured. Internal versus contract manufacturing, multiple plants with differing manufacturing equipment, and sources of raw material supply and specialized testing equipment are all requirements that need to be considered by the formulator in order to provide counsel to the supply-chain groups involved with the decision.

6.17.6 STABILITY

Formula

Preliminary formulas that may become candidates for finalization should undergo some degree of accelerated temperature stability testing in order for the formulator to determine if formulation or processing changes will be made to ensure formula stability.

These "informal" stabilities are usually conducted in glass bottles or jars and have a condensed stability protocol. Typically, samples will be placed at 45°C, Ambient (25°C), 5°C, and perhaps Freeze/Thaw cycling and exposure to sunlight, if product is clear or packaging is transparent. Observations are usually made weekly for approximately four weeks to assess overall formula stability. At this point, the formulator is looking for separation, discoloration, excessive changes in viscosity (that can be seen by observing product movement in package), malodor formation, etc. These stability evaluations are simply tools to help the formulator determine what may need to be done through the formula finalization process and are not used to ensure ultimate formula stability.

Alcohol-containing products or formula bases for pressurized packaging have specialized stability test packaging and may require special ovens or containers for accelerated temperature testing.

Formula in Package

If the final packaging or a similar package (material of construction) is available, samples should be placed on the same informal stability evaluation as the glass samples above. This will provide the formulator with information regarding gross interactions between the product and primary package.

Microbiology

Initial prototype development should include the preservative system identified for the formula/product of interest. Initial prototypes should undergo microbiological testing (initial total plate count and efficacy of preservation testing) to ensure that the preservative system is adequate to be carried through the remainder of the development process. Most organizations have a protocol for microbiological testing, and there are other protocols available through professional and regulatory groups (e.g., Personal Care Products Council).

Cost

Formula costs should be determined on preliminary prototypes to ensure compliance with the targets established at the onset of a project. Some organizations have protocols established for this early costing; otherwise, the formulator should independently calculate the approximate cost of prototypes using the standard costs or supplier costs provided for the raw materials contained in the prototype formulas.

Patent Status

The legal group should be provided key initial prototype formulations in order to obtain Freedom to Practice clearance or to determine if a new invention process should be initiated.

Selecting Final Prototype(s)

During the initial prototype development phase, a primary prototype(s) will be identified. These prototypes will successfully meet all of the evaluations conducted in the preliminary phase or result from modifications made at that time. It is at this point that the formulator needs to be very objective in evaluations. Forgiving prototype failures early on will eventually cause significant problems in finalizing the formula.

6.17.7 PERSONAL TRIAL

Dispensing from Package

The formulator should spend time simply dispensing the product from the package and dispensing mechanism established for the product. Observing product being dispensed into the hand or on a substrate similar to the substrate for which it is intended will provide the formulator with the information required to determine if formula should remain a viable candidate.

Aesthetics

The formulator should critically evaluate the aesthetic properties of the leading candidate formulas before, during, and after stability testing. Color, clarity, emulsion appearance, etc. should all be reviewed. If the formulator has any doubts regarding objectivity, other formulators or colleagues can be asked to provide an unbiased opinion.

Performance

If at all possible, the formulator should personally try the leading prototype(s) to develop a sense of the ultimate consumer experience. Other formulators and colleagues can also be enlisted to try the prototypes and offer their opinions/comments regarding the performance.

If there are safety issues related to using the products, or if the products are of a reactive nature (e.g., color), the formulator can use the product on artificial substrates (e.g., human hair) to determine how the prototype applies, is worked through, rinses out, and the final feel and/or appearance of the substrate.

6.17.8 PRELIMINARY STABILITY

Glass and Package of Interest

Prior to selecting the primary prototype(s), the formulator should critically review all of the stability information from the informal stabilities in glass and, if available, in packaging approximating the final product primary package. Again, it is critically important for the formulator to remain as objective as possible regarding the formula stability. If necessary, small batches of the primary prototype(s) should be prepared and the stability repeated, at least in glass. Any changes in processing parameters on these small batches should be diligently recorded to be used in developing the final manufacturing process. Again, having other formulators or colleagues offer their opinions on the stabilities can help the formulator remain unbiased.

Microbiology

All results related to the microbiological integrity of the primary prototype(s) and the efficacy of the selected preservative system in any of the prototypes tested should be reviewed. Special attention should be paid to the adequacy of preservation testing.

Pilot Scale Manufacturing/Filling

The primary prototype(s) should now be manufactured at a pilot scale. Some organizations have process engineering groups to perform this function, other organizations leave this to the manufacturing group, and still others leave this responsibility with the formulation group. Regardless, it is important to test the manufacture of the formula at a larger scale. Mixing, heating, and cooling rates, etc. are all different with scale, and those differences can have significant impact on the type and stability of final product, especially in the cases of emulsions. Filling can also impact the final aesthetics of the formula, so final prototype(s) should be filled by a method that approximates final filling operations as closely as possible.

Product manufactured at this small-scale level can and should be used for a complete stability test (glass and package) at all of the organizationally required conditions. These should include 45°C, 35°C, Ambient (25°C), 5°C, Freeze/Thaw (at least three and preferably five cycles), and exposure to sunlight. Stability should include sensory evaluation (appearance, odor, color), physical measurement (e.g., viscosity), chemical measurements (pH and active ingredients, if applicable), and microbiological testing (TPC and Challenge testing) at least at three and six months during the stability evaluation. Organizational stability protocols should be followed but should include evaluations at two weeks, one month, three months, six months, and one year at a minimum, with most protocols requiring an additional evaluation at two years, at least at ambient conditions.

Cost Verification

The formula cost of the final prototype(s) should be verified at this point. New raw material costs should be confirmed and whatever costs related to the formula should be included. Small-scale pilot manufacture may provide manufacturing cost estimates. The formulator should be aware of all of the costs, but is most concerned with the actual formulation costs.

Small-Scale Consumer Testing

Product from the pilot-scale manufacturing can be used for small-scale consumer testing if possible. Some degree of safety testing or review and approval is usually required prior to exposing formulas to consumers. Various organizations have different ways of conducting small-scale consumer testing—some have dedicated groups to recruit consumers, place products, and gather and analyze data, some place this testing through consumer research organizations that handle all of the administration and reporting, and some organizations use employee panels for this testing. This testing should be done to ensure acceptable product performance prior to more expensive and complex, large-scale consumer testing or actual marketing of product.

Claims Review/Testing

With the selection of final prototypes, claims testing should begin in earnest. All serious primary prototypes should be tested, as well as controls. This testing may involve the use of existing or published claims methods (e.g., diastron tensile strength testing), require the development of new testing methodologies, or use expert consumers or large-scale consumer testing to support claims.

No matter what the testing methodology is, a plan should be developed that specifically lists all of the claims to be made and the methodology to be used to provide the support. Some claims may be supported by a simple written document (e.g., "contains" claims). Other claims will require significant testing. It has been said that "extraordinary claims require extraordinary support." All parties involved with the claim development, support, and approval (Formulation, Marketing, Legal/Regulatory) should review and approve the claims support plan.

6.17.9 FINAL FORMULATION

Large-Scale Manufacturing and Filling

Once the final formulation has been identified, a large-scale production batch should be manufactured and filled to finalize manufacturing procedure and to provide "real world" samples for consumer testing, final stability testing, final microbiological testing, final claims testing, and if required, final safety testing.

This large-scale batch should use all of the equipment that is expected to be used in routine manufacture. This will provide the formulator with information to finalize finished formula specifications and provide confidence that the formula that will ultimately move into the consumer's hands exhibits all of the properties desired by the formulator.

Cost Verification

The large-scale manufacturing/filling trial will provide information related to the final overall cost of the product. While the formulator is really most concerned with the formula cost, all of the costs that go into a product can impact the total formula cost permitted.

6.17.10 FINAL STABILITY

Formula

Accelerated stability testing should be conducted on samples from the large-scale manufacturing trial. Most organizations have a stability protocol, but this should include 45°C, 35°C, Ambient (25°C), 5°C, F/T (at least three cycles), and exposure to sunlight. The formula should test samples taken from the batch prior to filling (in glass) along with the filled samples. This will identify any stability issues created by the pumping and filling process. Samples used in the final stability evaluation should be in glass (for observation) and in the final package, to be used for other testing (e.g., viscosity measurement).

Packaging

If the package has been labeled or decorated, the formulator may want to test the effect of product on the label or decoration. This particular testing may be conducted by a separate group (Packaging), but it should be completed on these samples.

Microbiological Integrity

Total plate count on adequacy of preservation testing should be conducted on samples obtained before the transfer/filling operation and also on samples that have gone through the entire filling operation. This will provide the formulator with confidence that the formula can withstand the rigors of normal production, from a microbiological integrity perspective.

Safety Testing

If required, safety testing or evaluation can be conducted on samples obtained from the large-scale manufacturing/filling trial.

Large-Scale Consumer Testing

Samples from the large-scale manufacturing/filling test can be used for large-scale consumer testing, if required. Once organizational product safety requirements have been met, samples may be placed with a large number of consumers (n = 300) to obtain final information related to consumer satisfaction. These tests are usually conducted by organizations whose specific function is to conduct consumer testing. This testing may require undecorated packaging, so the formulator needs to be aware of all requirements for this testing.

PART 6.18

ORAL CARE: FORMULATING PRODUCTS AND PRACTICES FOR HEALTH AND BEAUTY

By

Caren M. Barnes
Professor Coordinator of Clinical Research
University of Nebraska Medical Center College of Dentistry

Chi Shing Wong
Member, Product Development Group
Colgate-Palmolive Global Toothbrush Division

James G Masters, Ph.D.
Director in the Research and Development Division
Colgate-Palmolive Company

Shira Pilch, Ph.D.
Associate Director: Research and Development Division
Colgate-Palmolive Company

Michael Prencipe, Ph.D.
Director in the Research and Development Division
Colgate-Palmolive Company

ABSTRACT

The desire to have a beautiful smile with glistening white teeth is a universal aspiration, as important to the aesthetic sense as having a youthful, wrinkle-free skin or a beautifully sculpted body. This article highlights the importance of this area to both the dental profession and the consumer, and discusses the growing demand for aesthetic dental procedures.

Having a beautiful smile involves more than brushing one's teeth twice a day. For generations, the mouth was not considered to have an effect on total body health, nor was the mouth considered to reflect total body health. The relationship of total body health and oral health is explained in this chapter. However, it is clear that total body health includes having a state of oral health. Current issues around oral health are also discussed, such as the effects of aging on oral health.

This chapter contains scientific, evidence-based information on daily oral health regimes that are thorough and effective, including proper brushing, cleaning between teeth, and techniques for resolving halitosis. The key to a healthy mouth is the thorough, daily removal of dental plaque biofilm that must be performed mechanically, whether with a manual or powered toothbrush and with some method of removing the dental plaque biofilm from the surfaces of the tongue and between the teeth.

The chapter contains detailed information (i.e., ingredients, design) about oral hygiene products necessary for achieving and maintaining oral health. The oral hygiene products encompassed are toothpastes, mouthrinses, manual and powered toothbrushes, and waterflossers (Waterpik) as well as products for cleaning surfaces between the teeth and the ingredients that make them effective for specific oral problems, such as inflamed gums (gingivitis), cavities (dental caries), removal of dental stains and/or whitening teeth, and treatment of hypersensitivity.

TABLE OF CONTENTS

6.18 INTRODUCTION

A. Important Issues in Oral Health

Dental Plaque Biofilm

The role of dental plaque biofilm has been recognized for decades as being the agent responsible for dental caries and periodontal disease. Through ongoing research it is now recognized that dental plaque biofilm has a potential, if not definitive role, in the link between systemic and oral diseases. Dental plaque biofilm consists of over 500 species of bacteria that live in a well-organized bacterial community and are embedded in an extracellular slime layer that adheres to the surface of teeth and soft oral tissues. The links between dental plaque biofilm and systemic disease are related to the magnitude of the number of bacteria that reside in dental plaque biofilm as well as the inflammatory conditions they set up in the oral cavity and become involved with other parts of the body and thus, systemic disease. Research on the links between systemic and oral diseases have been and continue to be heavily researched.

Dental Caries

The past 50 years have seen a shift in what has previously been considered "oral" health. The shift has been from a focus on teeth and gingiva to the realization, by multiple healthcare professions, that the mouth is a mirror of the state of health or disease in individuals.[1] Great strides have been made in the past fifty years in the reduction of the prevalence of dental caries, although this is clearly still a significant public health issue. Clearly, fluoride is effective when delivered from toothpaste and incorporated in drinking water. By this means dental caries rates have decreased 30–50%.[2] Fluoridated water supplies in the U.S. have saved more than $4.6 billion annually in dental costs.[2] On a community level, the Centers for Disease Control and Prevention have reported that for every dollar spent on water fluoridation, $7.00–$42.00 is saved in oral health treatment costs, depending on the size of the community.[2] Assessments to determine risk for dental caries are being utilized (Caries Assessment and Management By Risk Assessment: CAMBRA), and notably there have been advancements in dental caries detection devices, particularly with the use of digital radiographs, quantitative light fluorescence, and fiber optic trans-illumination along with other new caries detection devices.[3] For over a decade we have had the scientific evidence that dental sealants do work, particularly those applied to children in school programs.[4] In addition, fluoride varnishes are playing an ever-increasing major role in the fight against cavities due to their proven efficacy and ease of application at the dentist office.

Periodontal Disease

The success for preventing periodontal disease has not been as effective as it has for dental caries. The results of a major study, Prevalence of Periodontitis in Adults in the United States: 2009 and 2010 estimates that 47.2%, or 64.7 million American adults, have some form of periodontal disease. Gingivitis, an inflammation of the gingiva, can be reversed; periodontitis cannot. If gingivitis is left untreated, inflammation can progress from the gingiva and will begin to affect the supporting structures of the teeth. The bone that supports the tooth in the affected socket(s) will be destroyed as well as the fibers that connect the root of the teeth to the bone.

Periodontal disease can be stopped most times with appropriate professional treatment and diligent homecare by the patient but the destruction, for the most part, cannot be reversed. Periodontal disease can be mild, moderate or severe, is a cumulative disease and, in adults 65 and older, its prevalence rate (evidence of having had period at some point in their lives) increases to 70.1 percent as described in a study published in the *Journal of Dental Research*, the official publication of the International and American Associations for Dental Research.

Currently there is ongoing research on oral changes that occur due to systemic diseases, access to oral care initiatives, and studies of the effects of aging on the oral cavity. There is no doubt at this time that a focus will remain on prevention and treatment of dental caries and periodontal disease.[5] It is also strongly believed there will continue to be research on oral cancer and the links between systemic diseases such as diabetes and the state of health or disease of the oral cavity as well as the effect that they have upon each other. The Centers for Disease Control and Prevention's Oral Health Program is currently developing new Strategic Planning for 2015 and several years beyond. Notably, some of their priority areas in their strategic planning include, but are not limited to study of: dental caries, periodontal diseases, oral and pharyngeal (mouth and throat) cancers, infection control, and elimination of health disparities.

In addition to dental caries and periodontal disease there are some other topics that are of paramount interest to both patients and dental health care providers. These topics include:

- Aesthetic dentistry,
- Halitosis (bad breath), and
- Oral issues related to aging.

Since this is a chapter in a book on Beauty and Health, we call particular attention to these latter subjects, for they are the quintessential focus of the aging population's search to look good and feel good in their advancing years. We are all concerned, no matter our age, with how we look, and healthy white teeth that can be used to chew what we like is a fundamental quest for all.

B. Importance of Aesthetics in Dentistry

The importance of an individual's appearance for aesthetic reasons is easy to assess, even if one did nothing but look at the sales of tooth-whitening agents. Americans spent approximately $1.4 billion on over-the-counter whitening agents in 2013.[6] Every four years the American Academy of Cosmetic Dentistry (AACD) conducts a survey of its membership. The most widely read one, the Cosmetic Dentistry State of the Industry 2011 Survey,[7] was distributed to AACD members in 2011 and had a response rate of 76% (only AACD members received the survey). Table 1 contains a list of the percentage of aesthetic procedures performed by AACD members, which these dentists have reported as distinctly not essential restorative procedures. As seen in Table 1, 85 to 95% of the procedures performed by these dentists are very expensive and procedures performed strictly for aesthetic reasons are few and far between since they are generally not covered by dental insurance.

Another interesting factor that resulted from analysis of the AACD 2011 survey responses is that the results indicated what the patients in these cosmetic practices really cared about most in terms of the cosmetic dentistry they received. The factor that was listed as the most important one, by 97% of the respondents, was appearance.

Table 1. Percent of esthetic procedures performed by members of the American Academy of Cosmetic Dentistry in 2010.[8]

COSMETIC PROCEDURES	PERCENT OF PROCEDURES PERFORMED IN 2010 BY AACD MEMBER SURVEY RESPONDENTS
Crown and bridge	95
Bleaching/ whitening	91
Direct bonding: Anterior	90
Veneers	85
Removable Prosthetics	84
Implants	83
Direct bonding: Posterior	83
Inlays or Onlays	67
Other cosmetic procedures	54
Orthodontics	54

C. Halitosis (oral malodor)

Along with appearance, having halitosis or bad breath is of great concern by the public. According to a popular Internet dating source[9] it is estimated that in the U.S., people spent approximately \$10 billion dollars per year on mouthwashes, breath mints, rinses, gum, toothpastes and other products to treat or mask halitosis. Specifically, in 2011–2012, people in the U.S. spend approximately \$1.6 billion per year on toothpaste and \$1.43 billion on toothbrushes and dental accessories such as interdental cleaners and dental floss. *These statistics provide insight as to how important appearance and alleviation of bad breath (and oral health) is to individuals and how much money they are willing to spend on their appearance and to have fresh breath.*

Before halitosis can be alleviated, the source of the bad breath needs to be detected. The source may be related to a systemic disease or problem—or, it can have origins in the oral cavity. If the oral cavity is not suspected as the source for the halitosis, the patient should be referred to a physician for evaluation of body systems. Non-oral sources for halitosis[10, 11] include:

- Nasal cavity
- Nasopharyngeal areas
- Sinuses
- Oropharyngeal areas
- Lung

- Lower respiratory tract
- Systemic diseases
- Gastrointestinal diseases and disorders
- Foods, fluids, and medications

However, 80–90% of halitosis originates in the oral cavity.[12–14] Halitosis is classified into categories of genuine halitosis, pseudo-halitosis, and halitophobia. Genuine halitosis is further classified as pathogenic halitosis or physiologic halitosis. Pathogenic halitosis is further classified as oral and extra-oral halitosis, indicating that the halitosis has its origin in the oral cavity or outside the oral cavity. Patients with pseudo-halitosis and halitophobia complain about oral halitosis that does not exist. Dental healthcare providers are equipped to work with individuals who have pseudo-halitosis, but halite-phobic patients may need psychiatric treatment.

Halitosis is best measured by gas chromatography analysis. Gas chromatography is specific for identifying the concentration of volatile sulfur compounds, which is the cause of most oral malodors.[10] Individuals with periodontal disease and halitosis would have their halitosis classified as pathogenic in that it results from the bacteria involved in periodontal disease. When patients have periodontal pockets of 4 mm or more, volatile sulfuric compounds are released and responsible for halitosis.

Patients with xerostomia, or dry mouth, may have halitosis, since bacteria and oral debris are not physiologically washed away as they normally would be during routine cleaning of the mouth. Giving patients with xerostomia salivary substitutes can help the halitosis if the teeth are kept as free as possible from dental plaque and the tongue is cleaned on a regular basis. Dental hygienists and dentists are poised to address the reasons for halitosis that are oral related. If a patient mentions halitosis, the dental hygienist needs to include the halitosis as something that needs to be addressed in the treatment plan. The dental hygienist can work individually with each patient to show them how to best remove the dental plaque and debris from their mouth and what products to use. This approach can be effective in helping patients prevent halitosis; if the patient does practice thorough oral hygiene and still has halitosis, he may need to be referred to medical personnel for further evaluation.

Mouthrinses and breath mints can be effective in masking some oral malodors, but usually these products have to be used repeatedly every few hours unless they have antimicrobial properties. Halitosis can be resolved in some patients with through regular dental plaque removal utilizing a toothbrush and a method for cleaning between the teeth. If dental floss is too narrow to touch the surfaces of both teeth when placed between them, then dental floss needs to be discarded and a new method of interdental cleaning should be utilized. One alternative in such cases is the use of interdental brushes. These come in several sizes and shapes and the brushes that can fill the interdental space will most likely remove the most dental plaque and biofilm.[15]

Patients will use a variety of products to fight oral malodor, in addition to using a toothbrush and interdental cleaning device. Mouthrinses that are antimicrobial such as chlorhexidine may be useful for neutralizing volatile sulfur-containing compounds. Table 2 contains a list of ingredients used to fight oral malodor and can be found in mouthrinses, toothpastes, breath mints, and chewing gum.

Table 2. List of active ingredients used to fight oral malodor and how they work to alleviate oral malodor

ACTIVE INGREDIENTS USED TO FIGHT ORAL MALODOR	ACTION AGAINST ORAL MALODOR
Chlorhexidine	Antimicrobial; neutralizes volatile sulfuric compounds
Cetylpridinium chloride Triclosan Essential oils	Mild antimicrobial Agent affecting volatile sulfuric compound producing microorganisms
Chlorine dioxide Zinc	Volatile sulfuric compound neutralizing agent

D. Oral Issues Related to Aging

1. Demographics of Aging: What to Expect

There is a burgeoning population of people aged 65 years and over in the United States. They are generally described as the "Baby Boomers." These individuals represent the post-World War II generation born between the years of 1946 and 1964. In the year 2010, the "Baby Boomers" began turning age 65 and with this tipping point a new market emerged focused on the needs of these aging citizens. The growth of the population of those 65 years and over has many societal effects as the needs of these aging individuals have to be met. This growth of numbers of the aging population will have an increasingly significant effect on healthcare providers, businesses, families, and policymakers at all levels of government. It is important to be familiar with some of the "facts" related to this expanding group of aging citizens.[16]

- In 2010, there were 40 million people age 65 and over who represented 13 percent of the total U.S. population; by the year 2030, 20 percent of all Americans will be age 65 or older.
- After 2030, the growth rate of the group of individuals 65 and over is projected to remain at a steady 20 percent.

- After 2030, the "Baby Boomers" will enter the "oldest-old population" (those 85 and over), causing this group to grow rapidly.
- In 2010, the population of those aged 85 years and over was 5.5 million. By 2050, the U.S. Census Bureau projects that the "oldest-old population" will grow to 19 million. Further, there are some research projections that predict that the death rates of the "oldest-old population" may decline at a more rapid rate than is predicted by the U.S. Census Bureau.

2. Oral Health and the Aging

The current U.S. population of aging seniors has enjoyed unprecedented advances in oral hygiene and greater access to dental treatment than previous generations. Some of the advances they have benefited from include:

- Availability of over-the-counter fluoridated toothpaste (1955) and water fluoridation
- Availability of dental insurance in the (1970s)
- *U.S. dental healthcare providers embraced the concept of preventing dental disease* rather than treating the consequences of common dental diseases. Increasingly an expanded focus has been generated in the areas of dental caries and emphasis has been placed on plaque-control programs with individualized oral hygiene instructions for patients (late 1960s and early 1970s)
- Dental sealants (1974), fluoride varnishes, and high-fluoride toothpastes (1980s)

As a result of these advances, the majority of current seniors have all or most of their teeth.[17] This presents a unique problem when these seniors enter hospitals, nursing homes, and long-term care facilities. Nursing care staff are presented with having to provide or assist these seniors with brushing and related oral hygiene procedures. Nursing staff are now required to do much more than "scrub" dentures in a sink.

Certainly not all senior citizens reside in nursing homes or long-term care facilities. There is a distinct difference between the type of oral health issues senior citizens face, depending on whether they are living independently or live in a facility where they must depend on assistance with oral hygiene procedures. There are some oral health issues that seniors face no matter where they live and are congruent with the normal aging process. Some of the normal signs of aging that can be observed in the oral cavity of those over 65 years of age can be seen in Table 3.

Dental examinations and professional cleaning of the teeth are as important during the senior years of life as they have been through the previous stages of life. Dentists and dental hygienists can find early signs of problems and take measures to help the patient halt damage and prevent greater damage. There are

Table 3. Clinical Signs Of Aging And The Associated Cause[18]

CLINICAL SIGN OF AGING IN THE ORAL CAVITY	APPEARANCE IN THE ORAL CAVITY	CAUSE
Dry lips, tongue and inside of the oral cavity; rapidly progressing tooth decay	The smooth surfaces inside the oral cavity will appear dry and normal elasticity is not present; smooth tissue surfaces as well as gingiva will be red and inflamed; large amounts of dental plaque will accumulate at the gum line of the teeth. Teeth may experience rapid tooth decay due to the loss of the cleansing effect of saliva. Swallowing may be difficult.	Diminished salivary gland flow; can be caused as a result of normal aging or as a result of the effects of medication. This condition is known as xerostomia. There are over 800 medications that can cause xerostomia or dry mouth.
Recession of the gingiva	Teeth will appear to have a "longer appearance" as the gingiva recedes	Gingiva may recede as a normal part of aging; can be a sign of periodontal disease; 75% of seniors have some form of periodontal disease
Erosion, attrition of the teeth, dental decay	Flattening of the chewing surfaces of the teeth; notches in the enamel at the gum line of the tooth; teeth may be hypersensitive and the patient may react to pain when ingesting sugary foods or food that is hot or cold	Wearing of tooth structure due to chewing. Can occur due to abnormal alignment of teeth, repeated exposure to acid from foods or acidic drinks; lack of removal of dental plaque (bacteria) on a daily basis and/or lack of professional cleaning and fluoride treatments.
Mobile teeth	May appear normal but during chewing the tooth or teeth are loose.	Bone loss and loss of fibers holding the tooth in the socket due to periodontal disease
Stained teeth	Teeth may have a yellow, gray or brown discoloration of the teeth.	Smoking, coffee and tea stains, natural process of aging; dentinal tubules are filled with minerals and the teeth take on a yellowed or gray appearance

medications and products that are especially formulated to alleviate some of the symptoms of dry mouth. Professional fluoride applications in the form of fluoride treatments with trays or fluoride varnish can provide relief from hypersensitivity and the softening of enamel due to the acidic destruction process that occurs with the dental decay process.

Dental healthcare professionals can recommend dentifrices that are specially formulated, for example to prevent or stop decay, stop hypersensitivity, or whiten teeth. Therefore, it is important for dental hygienists and dentists to stay abreast of advancements made with various oral care products, new benefits, and the ingredients they are formulated with. In this way they can guide their patients to the most appropriate dentifrice to meet their patient's needs. Table 4 contains a list of popular ingredients found in dentifrices and their functions.

Table 4. Basic Ingredients in Dentifrices[21]

INGREDIENT	AMOUNT	PURPOSE	SPECIFIC INGREDIENTS
Abrasives	20-40%	Clean and polish	Calcium carbonate, silicone oxides, aluminum oxide, calcium pyrophosphate
Binders	2%	Prevents separation of ingredients	Alginate, synthetic cellulose, gums
Coloring agents	2%	Attractive appearance	Vegetable dyes
Detergents	1-2%	Foaming action; helps loose debris	Sodium lauryl sulfate, sodium lauryl sarcosinate
Flavoring agents		Pleasant taste that is a lingering aftertaste	Essential oils: peppermint, spearmint, wintergreen, cinnamon, menthol
Preservatives	<1%	Prevent growth of bacteria and mold	Sodium benzoate, alcohols, dichlorinated phenols
Sweeteners	2%	Pleasant flavor	Saccharine, sorbitol, mannitol, xylitol, glycerin
Water and humectants	20-40%	Maintain moisture and consistency	Sorbitol, glycerin, propylene glycol, mannitol

6.18.1 PERSONAL ORAL CARE

The number and type of oral care products available for personal oral care is unprecedented. Notably, there is a vast range of prices, making some of these oral care products affordable for most everyone. In 2013, $1.8 billion was spent on dentifrices and spent $775 million on toothbrushes.[18, 19] There are many additional products that consumers use for oral care. These include but are not limited to products such as dental floss, interdental products for cleaning between teeth, mouthrinses, tongue cleaners (tongue cleaning is critically important to controlling halitosis), fluoride-containing products, antibacterial mouthrinses, waterflossers such as the Water-Pik, sonic devices that pulse water between teeth, and whitening products.

It is important for dental hygienists and dentists to be familiar with the various products so that when recommending a product to a patient, they can recommend the one that best fits the patient's needs. In this Internet age, it is also important for consumers to be knowledgeable about personal oral care products as well. Otherwise, they may make purchases of products that are ineffective or not appropriate for meeting their needs. A review of dental products is important so that patients and dental healthcare providers are knowledgeable about new developments in oral care products and especially the results of research findings about the efficacy of personal oral care products. Clinical research and systematic reviews have played a crucial role in revealing which products and ingredients are the most effective.

A. Dentifrices

One of the most common questions that dental hygienists and dentists are asked by patients is, "What brand of toothpaste should I use?" Most often, the response from the dental healthcare professional will be based on the patient's needs. The conditions that are considered when professionally recommending a dentifrice are prevention of dental caries and/or the demineralization/erosion of enamel, gingivitis and/or periodontal disease, sensitivity, or stained teeth. Additionally, dental healthcare professionals most often recommend dentifrices that have the Seal of Acceptance from the American Dental Association: http://www.ada.org/en/public-programs/ada-seal-of-acceptance-program/.

1. Regulation (Therapeutic vs. Cosmetic Benefits)

The American Dental Association awards its Seal of Acceptance to dental products based on a review of: (1) the data supporting a product's efficacy and safety, and (2) the claims made for the product, to ensure that all claims are supported by the science. Application for the American Dental Association's Seal of Acceptance is strictly voluntary and manufacturers submit their dentifrices to the American Dental Association for testing and review. Dentists and dental hygienists need to be familiar with the wide array of dentifrices so they can guide their patients to the most appropriate dentifrice that is safe and effective and meet their needs.

It is important to note that the U.S. Food and Drug Administration regulates dentifrices under the Federal Food, Drug and Cosmetic Act. The FDA sets standards on dentifrice effectiveness and safety and regulates the amount and type of ingredients that can be in a dentifrice formulation. Table 4 contains information about the ingredients common to most dentifrice formulations regulated by the FDA.

Dentifrices are considered by the FDA to be a drug, as most dentifrices contain fluoride to prevent tooth decay or specific ingredients to treat sensitivity and gingivitis, among others. Therapeutic agents are by definition concerned with the treatment of disease. Cosmetics, as defined by the U.S. Food and Drug Administration, are "intended to be applied to the human body for cleansing, beautifying, promoting attractiveness, or altering the appearance without affecting the body's structure or functions."

2. Stain Removal

Dentifrices, along with toothbrushes, are the most widely used and recommended oral products. Dentifrices have been used to freshen breath since the time of the Greeks and Romans, and have usually included abrasive agents to help remove stain. Dentifrices alone, however, will not remove dental plaque and biofilm. At this time, dental plaque must be mechanically removed. Use of dentifrices adds the benefit of containing abrasive agents that help with the mechanical removal of dental plaque and stain (thus also providing whitening efficacy) and most are flavored with the intent to freshen breath.

3. Abrasion

Another important fact that dental hygienists and dentists need to be aware of is the abrasiveness of dentifrices. There are several issues that need to be addressed when a dental hygienist or dentist recommends a dentifrice to a patient: whether the patient needs a dentifrice 1) with fluoride for dental caries prevention and/or control, 2) with antimicrobial medications for the prevention and control of gingivitis, 3) sensitivity ingredients to control dentinal hypersensitivity, and 4) with odor-controlling ingredients to manage halitosis. Another issue is the type of restorations and restorative materials that are in the patient's mouth—especially aesthetic-restorative materials. Aesthetic-restorative materials, which include several types of tooth-colored materials, can be easily damaged with highly abrasive dentifrices.

Dentifrice abrasiveness has traditionally been determined by the Relative Dentin Abrasivity Index (RDA), a standardized test developed by the American Dental Association. One should note there are many other factors that affect the impact toothbrushing can have on hard and soft tissues, such as type of brush used (soft, medium, hard bristles), consumer habits, etc., and one should not put too much emphasis on any single factor. The maximum recommended RDA value for toothpastes is set at 250.

The abrasives used in dentifrices help remove dental plaque and stains from the tooth surface. An ideal abrasive level of a dentifrice would provide the ability to clean the tooth surfaces and remove stains without causing damage to the tooth surface or to the surface of dental restorations. The Council on Dental Therapeutics of the American Dental Association states that "a dentifrice should be no more abrasive than is necessary to keep the teeth clean—that is, free of accessible plaque, debris, and superficial stain. The degree of abrasivity needed to accomplish this purpose may vary from one individual to another."

The abrasivity and cleaning action of abrasives are related to abrasive particle size, shape, brittleness, and hardness. The most commonly used abrasives are: hydrated silica, calcium carbonate, calcium pyrophosphate, and dicalcium phosphate dihydrate. Other materials include sodium bicarbonate, tricalcium phosphate, sodium metaphosphate, and alumina or aluminum hydroxide.

4. Ingredients

Dentists and dental hygienists need to be familiar with the wide array of dentifrices and their ingredients so they can guide their patients to the most appropriate dentifrice to meet their needs. For example, a patient may want to know what the best whitening dentifrice to buy is, but the dental hygienist has taken note that this patient has dentinal hypersensitivity. A whitening dentifrice containing hydrogen peroxide or carbamide peroxide or a dentifrice that is highly abrasive would all be contraindicated for this patient as these types of dentifrices could worsen the dentinal hypersensitivity.

Table 5 contains a list of popular active ingredients found in dentifrices and the conditions they are intended to target. Adding active ingredients is not easily accomplished, as many potential actives can interact or react with the other ingredients. Interactions between potential therapeutic agents and inactive ingredients are well covered in a separate review.[20]

Abrasives. *Hydrated silica* (or silica as it is sometimes called) has become the most widely used abrasive in the United States and many other countries over the last 25 years. Hydrated silica used as an abrasive is manufactured by either gelation or precipitation. A xerogel is manufactured by drying the gel formed by gelation with subsequent milling to obtain the desired particle size. The precipitates are collected and dried. Use of these hydrated silica abrasives is the basis for clear gel toothpastes; their use is practical in opacified gel toothpastes as well. The advantages in using hydrated silicas as abrasives include: a high degree of compatibility with fluoride salts, flavors, and other materials, as well as higher efficiency in cleaning tooth surfaces as compared to most other toothpaste abrasives.

Table 5. List of popular ingredients in dentifrices and the functions they serve.

ACTIVE INGREDIENT	PURPOSE
Calcium carbonate	Remineralization
Carbamide peroxide	Whitening agent for bleaching teeth
Humectants, lubricants, enzymes, polymers	Alleviate symptoms of xerostomia (dry mouth); helps to retain moisture in oral soft tissues such as the inside of the cheeks and lips
Hydrogen peroxide	Antibacterial; whitening agent for bleaching teeth
Potassium nitrate 5% (some dentifrices contain 5% potassium nitrate and fluoride	Desensitization; relieve hypersensitivity caused by exposed dentin; helps block sensations of pain
Pyrophosphates: sodium hexametaphosphate, tetrapotassium pyrophosphate; gantrez, zinc chloride, zinc citrate	Anticalculus capabilities; softens calculus making removal easier
Sodium bicarbonate	Neutralizes acids from dental plaque; very low abrasion, effectively removes stains, inhibits volatile sulfuric compounds to reduce oral malodor
Sodium fluoride	Works to strengthen enamel and helps prevent dental caries
Sodium monofluorophosphate	Works to strengthen enamel and helps prevent dental caries
Stannous fluoride	Works to remineralize enamel after dental caries attack helps to prevent root caries; anticaries, antiplaque and antigingivitis effects
Stannous fluoride (0454%) and sodium hexametaphosphate	Anticaries, antigingivitis, antiplaque, reduction of sensitivity and stain
Strontium chloride	Desensitization; relieve hypersensitivity caused by exposed dentin; helps block sensations of pain
Triclosan	Broad-spectrum antibacterial agent; antiplaque, antigingivitis and anti-inflammatory properties
Xylitol	Naturally occurring sugar substitute that has anticariogenic properties

Hydrated silica is available in many grades from various suppliers worldwide and ranges in abrasivity from fairly low to quite high. Common Particle Size Distributions used for abrasives range from about 5 to 35 microns. There also are dual-function hydrated silica grades available that also serve as toothpaste thickeners.

Calcium carbonate or chalk is available in a number of grades varying in crystalline form, particle size, and surface area. Precipitated calcium carbonate (PCC) is one of the earliest abrasives used and is still in use today, mainly due to its inherently low cost. Natural calcium carbonate is also available commercially and offers an even lower-cost option. Precipitated and natural calcium carbonate is sometimes used in combination to achieve optimal formulations in terms of cost and cleaning efficacy. All grades of calcium carbonate contain a finite amount of water-soluble calcium salts and will require compatible fluoride sources such as sodium monofluorophosphate. All calcium carbonate toothpastes are alkaline, and therefore they may also require flavors compatible at this higher pH.

Calcium phosphates include diverse chemicals, such as dicalcium phosphate dihydrate, dicalcium phosphate, tricalcium phosphate, calcium pyrophosphate, and synthetic apatites, all of which are used as toothpaste abrasives. *Dicalcium phosphate dihydrate* (DCP-D) is the calcium phosphate most commonly used in dentifrices. The pH of toothpaste made with DCP-D normally ranges from about 6 to 8. The taste of DCP-D-based toothpastes tends to be better than that of calcium carbonate–based products (not chalky), and flavor stability is usually less of a problem. DCP-D is in a metastable state and reverts to the anhydrous form with consequent hardening of the paste. This hardening is accelerated in the presence of fluoride ions and therefore DCP-D may be supplied with a stabilizer to delay or prevent this change. Trimagnesium phosphate, tetrasodium pyrophosphate, and other pyrophosphates are common stabilizers.

Calcium pyrophosphate (CPP) was originally developed as the abrasive of choice for products containing sodium or stannous fluoride. It is claimed that the low availability of soluble calcium ions contributes to the stability of the fluoride and this abrasive is experiencing a revival in whitening toothpastes such as Colgate Optic White™ (from Colgate-Palmolive) due to its inertness and excellent cleaning and polishing efficacy without corresponding higher dentine abrasivity.

Sodium bicarbonate or baking soda has been used as an abrasive in the United States since the early 1960s. Its drawbacks can be saltiness and high product pH, which may lead to some incompatibilities. It serves a second function because it can neutralize some odors in the mouth. In the United States, it has a mystique of being an odor reducer and a mild/gentle cleanser.

When recommending a dentifrice based on abrasivity, dental hygienists and dentists need to be certain that a patient received brushing instructions and does not brush too hard. A standard toothbrushing pressure is 150 grams of force (mass). If a patient is brushing in such a way that the bristles of the toothbrush are splayed outward, they likely are brushing much too hard. Figure 1 illustrates a toothbrush that has been used with too much force during brushing.

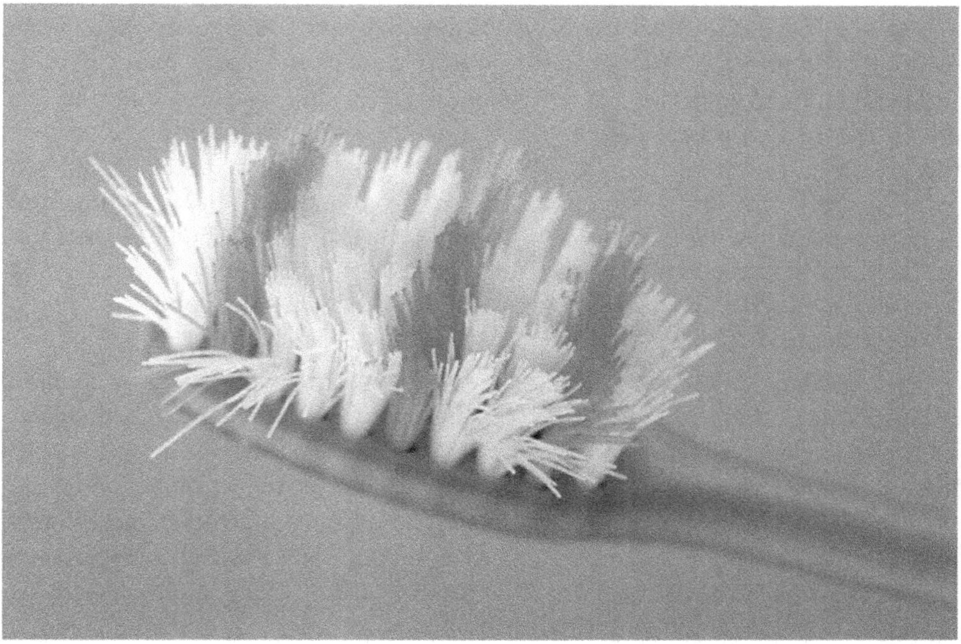

Figure 1. Toothbrush with splayed bristles caused from excessive brushing force. (Photo copyright by 123RF).

Humectants

It is necessary to incorporate a component with humectant properties to prevent toothpastes from drying out. This is most likely to happen if the cap is not replaced on the tube. Alternatively, if toothpaste is allowed to build up on the tube nozzle threads, the cap can become locked in place. An additional important factor is the enhanced and more pleasing "mouth-feel" achieved using the humectants listed below. *Glycerin* is the perfect humectant in that it is stable and nontoxic, has some solubilizing properties, contributes some sweetness and improves dentifrice mouth-feel. Today glycerin is available mostly in synthetic grades at 99% or higher levels. *Sorbitol* syrup 70% has been found useful since it has some properties similar to those of glycerin.

Propylene glycol has also been used as a component of the humectant system. The drawback here is that at high-usage levels it has a tendency to be somewhat bitter and is more costly than Sorbitol or Glycerin. *Xylitol* is manufactured from xylose and is noted for its pleasant coolness in the mouth when used at high levels. There are published studies supporting anti-caries properties, although U.S. regulations do not permit it to be claimed as an actual active ingredient in dentifrice products. While it is noticeably sweeter than sorbitol, it is also more expensive.

Polyethylene glycol or PEG is one of the dual-functional materials that can be used in toothpaste. The lower-molecular-weight materials, such as PEG-8, exhibit some humectant-like effects and act as lubricants to some degree and as processing aids to disperse some of the thickening agents that require hydration. In hydrated silica-based products even the low-molecular-weight PEGs act as thickening agents, with a more pronounced effect resulting from higher-molecular-weight PEGs up to PEG-20M. Problems related to their usage include the fact that the low-molecular-weight PEGs may be bitter and those higher in MW than PEG-18 require heat during processing in order to facilitate incorporation.

Water, which is used to provide semi-solid consistency, is a key ingredient and a critical component in dentifrice compositions, but also acts as a solubilizer for active agents such as the various forms of fluoride (neutral sodium fluoride, monosodium fluoride, stannous fluoride). Water is also included in most toothpaste intentionally due to its low cost and indirectly in other ingredients (some humectants contain 30% water). Keeping the overall water level low enough so as to prevent microbial growth is important. Measurements of water activity have been developed to help in formulating a microbiologically safe product without the need for using strong preservatives.

Surfactants

Tooth cleaning is partially a detergent-type process, and almost all toothpastes incorporate a surface-active agent. The ideal detergent should be tasteless, non-toxic, and nonirritant to the oral mucosa, while producing a large volume of dense but low expansion, foam with non-gagging qualities. Foam quality is important since it has a significant influence on the subjective assessment of toothpaste performance.

Sodium lauryl sulfate (SLS) is the most widely used detergent for oral products and satisfies almost all the requirements of the ideal detergent. In addition to sodium lauryl sulfate, various other detergents are also used.

Although not widely used, some other anionic detergents, i.e., *sodium methyl cocoyl taurate (tauranol)*, have found limited application in toothpaste. In addition, *poloxamer 407* and similar nonionic block copolymers have also been included in toothpaste formulations. Other types of foam boosters, such as cocoamidopropyl betaine, are zwitterionic.

Thickening and Binding Agents

A thickening or gelling agent is necessary in order to maintain the stability of a high-solids suspension. The thickening agent also modifies the dispersibility, foam character, and mouth-feel of dentifrices. Thickening agents used in toothpastes can be natural or synthetic gums that thicken when hydrated or inorganic materials such as hydrated silica or magnesium aluminum silicate.

Carrageenan is the generic name given to gums derived from the seaweed *Chondrus crispus* or Irish moss. Commercial carrageenans are standardized products of uniform and reproducible quality. This type of gum is rarely used by itself and is usually used in combination with others listed below.

Cellulose gum or sodium carboxymethyl cellulose (SCMC) comes in a variety of grades exhibiting different physical properties that may be controlled by adjusting the degree of breakdown of the cellulose before substitution, and by the degree of substitution. SCMC is reasonably stable in the presence of electrolytes and calcium ions and in general are suitable for most toothpaste formulations. Cellulose gum is the most commonly used gum for toothpastes. It imparts little color and is nontoxic and relatively tasteless. Due to its anionic nature, SCMC is not suitable for toothpastes containing cationic ingredients, especially certain antibacterials. For these pastes, nonionic cellulose derivatives such as *hydroxyethylcellulose* or *hydroxypropyl methylcellulose* may be used.

Xanthan gum is a bioengineered fermentation product that also finds application as a thickener in toothpaste and is widely used in the United States and elsewhere in toothpaste products. It might be the ideal thickener for toothpaste except for its relatively high cost.

Carbomer is available in various grades and has been used in toothpastes as a thickening agent. Thickening efficacy and utility depend on the pH and electrolyte content of the toothpaste, and therefore have limited utility and must usually be combined with other thickening agents to provide the necessary rheological properties necessary for consumer acceptable formulations, such as its stand-up.[20] The ideal toothpaste, from a rheological view, is one that is pseudoplastic and has a yield stress. This combination of properties allows the toothpaste to stay in the tube when the cap is off (high yield stress) but extrudable when the tube is squeezed (i.e., viscosity decreases with increasing stress; pseudoplastic).

Clays, in particular *magnesium aluminum silicate* and *sodium magnesium silicate*, continue to find usage as thickening agents in toothpaste.

Hydrated silica, discussed previously as an abrasive, exists in both gel and precipitated forms that are widely used as toothpaste thickeners. The average particle sizes used range from submicron to about 5 microns. Although both abrasive and thickening silicas are classified as hydrated silica, they differ in the degree to which these ingredients impart viscosity, which is dependent on porosity and structure properties of these raw materials.

Fumed or pyrogenic silica is rarely used, but offers significant advantages under conditions where high purity is required, such as in presence of reactive ingredients, i.e., oxidizing agents that can readily decompose in the presence of impurities often found in hydrated silicas. All forms of silica are highly compatible with fluorides and can yield a rapidly dispersing and highly consumer-acceptable toothpaste or gel. This type of silica is also useful as a thickener in toothpastes, especially in low-water or anhydrous compositions, where there is insufficient amount of water to properly hydrate the rheological additives listed above. It can be effective for this purpose, especially in conjunction with other polymers that are also effective in low-water systems.

Flavors. The perceived flavor of toothpaste is one of the most important characteristics influencing consumer acceptance. Consumers expect a clean mouth-feel after brushing and this is delivered in part by the flavor. Flavor also plays a large role in delivering fresh breath either by masking or modifying the perception of malodors. Flavor oils are usually the most expensive ingredients in toothpaste and can have the greatest impact on consumer acceptance, and are therefore created by experienced flavorists who tailor these for different regions of the globe.

In the United States, flavors have usually been based on spearmint, peppermint, and, to a smaller degree, wintergreen. Menthol is sometimes added, as are other cooling materials, to increase the cooling effect. Flavors can be modified with clove, eucalyptus, aniseed, cinnamon, and others. Other flavor modifiers such as woody, herbal, medicinal, and floral notes are used in different countries, and some are quite successful.

Various other ingredients of the toothpaste formulation can contribute to the perceived taste; for example, dicalcium phosphate dihydrate–based pastes usually have a taste preferred over those based on calcium carbonate. The hydrated silica–based toothpastes or gels are also noted for not having a significant taste impact. The flavor may also be modified by the presence of an active ingredient and even by the pH or electrolyte content of the product. The nature of the foam and the dispersibility of the paste can also modify flavor perception in the mouth. For these reasons, consumer acceptance of a given flavor should only be judged in the intended full base formulation and should be assessed in large consumer tests to ensure market success prior to launching of the product.

Colorants and Preservatives. Colors are often added to toothpastes, sometimes to mask an off-color from the base formulation either initially or upon storage. The range of colors available is restricted somewhat by food or drug additive regulations. In the United States, the predominantly used colorants are FD&C and D&C approved dyes and lakes, as well as a few allowable natural colorants.

Titanium dioxide is widely used in hydrated silica–based toothpastes as an opacifier and in other abrasive-system toothpastes to impart a bright white color to the products.

The range of toothpastes available today is quite varied. These can be opaque, white, or colored pastes, "water white" or colored clear gels, striped products, different-colored toothpastes, and gels delivered from two-compartment pumps or tubes. There are even products containing colored speckles composed of agglomerates of abrasive or speckles encapsulated by polymers and waxes. It is apparent that consumers have an interest in new visual effects in toothpaste products as well as by the mouth-feel delivered by the toothpaste, including particles that deliver a "dentist clean feel." There are also novel polymer systems to enhance the smoothness and thickness of foam generated by the surfactant systems such as those used in food industries as fat substitutes (i.e., microcrystalline cellulose).

The use of ***preservatives*** is becoming more common today as formulations are containing higher levels of water to reduce the overall cost of the product. *Sodium benzoate* is not very effective at neutral and higher pH values but is used fairly widely for in-process control of microorganisms. *Potassium sorbate* and the various *parabens* also find limited usage. Novel ingredients that are finding more applications as preservatives are select flavor components such as benzyl alcohol because of their efficacy, safety profile, and relatively low impact on taste. Products today are subjected to a battery of bacteriological challenge testing to ensure microbiological robustness during manufacture and consumer use.

5. Therapeutic Ingredients

Anti-Caries Agents. Fluoride ion delivered from a compatible toothpaste base has been shown in numerous clinical trials to reduce the incidence of carious lesions in both children and adults. It acts by reducing the acid solubility of tooth enamel. Fluoride has also been shown to aid in the remineralization of white-spot carious lesions.

Sodium fluoride, *sodium monofluorophosphate*, and *stannous fluoride* are the anti-caries actives of choice. In the United States the Final Monograph[21] defines the allowable levels of soluble fluoride ion from each salt in each allowable abrasive system for anti-caries active drugs. In a broad sense the only significant change from the earlier "accepted" target of 1000 ppm of fluoride is the addition of an allowable 1500 ppm of soluble fluoride ion from sodium fluoride and sodium monofluorophosphate. Also, since toothpaste is volume-dosed, the allowable level of total fluorine has been widened to 850–1150 to account for the varying specific gravities of toothpaste products. This document goes on to describe other test criteria that must be met, including enamel caries reduction, enamel solubility reduction, and fluoride uptake.[21] Any new agent would have to be approved by FDA through a rigorous process (New Drug Application, NDA) to determine safety and efficacy of the ingredient.

Actives for Prevention/Reduction of Plaque, Gingivitis, and Periodontitis

While most plaque control is achieved with mechanical removal such as proper and at least twice daily brushing and flossing, there is a significant portion of the population that suffers from gingivitis and periodontitis due to inadequate plaque removal, which occurs especially in hard-to-reach places. Therefore, addition of chemotherapeutic agents to oral care vehicles is necessary as an adjuvant to improve and enhance oral hygiene.

In the past two decades there have been significant advances in identifying and formulating antibacterial systems that are highly effective against plaque, gingivitis (a disease that can lead to redness and bleeding of gums), and periodontitis, which can eventually lead to tooth loss. Control of plaque especially at the gingival margin is then highly desirable in the maintenance of a healthy mouth.

Triclosan, a broad-spectrum, nonionic antibacterial agent, has been used by dentifrice manufacturers as a way to control plaque and gingivitis. A delivery system that can enhance the efficacy of triclosan is based on PVM/MA copolymer, which enhances the uptake of this antibacterial agent to hard and soft tissues in the mouth. Commercial toothpaste containing this active delivery system has been studied extensively for its safety and efficacy and has been granted the American Dental Association Seal of Acceptance for prevention against gingivitis, plaque, and cavities. It was also given approval for use in toothpastes by the U.S. Food and Drug Administration for prevention of gingivitis and cavities. Clinical studies have also shown the feasibility of prevention and control of periodontal disease using a chemotherapeutic dentifrice formulated with triclosan/copolymer system.[22]

There are other ingredients mentioned elsewhere in this chapter that have clinically demonstrated antiplaque and antigingivitis activity in either toothpaste or mouthrinses. These actives include *chlorhexidine* (mouthwash), *stannous fluoride* (toothpaste), *cetylpyridinium chloride* (mouthwash), and a mixture of phenolics and essential oils at specified levels (*thymol*, *eucalyptol*, *methyl salicylate*, and *menthol*) (mouthwash).

Other *herbal ingredients and extracts* have been reported to be active antiplaque and antigingivitis agents. Enzymes of various sorts have been used in toothpastes with claims for stain removal, whitening, antiplaque activity, and bad breath reduction. They can be denatured readily by some formulation ingredients such as anionic surfactants and temperature extremes and therefore create formulation problems.

Hypersensitivity

Dentin hypersensitivity is a common condition affecting up to 57% of adults, with highest incidence at age 30 and above. According to Brännström's hydrodynamic theory, tooth sensitivity[23] results when dentin tubule openings become exposed and fluid movement occurs as a result of tactile, chemical, evaporative, or osmotic stimuli. The fluid movement triggers mechano-receptors of pulpal nerve fibers and is interpreted by the brain as pain. Exposure of dentin commonly results from wearing away of the tooth's protective surfaces (cementum and enamel) due to gum recession, acid exposure, and/or abrasion. The management of dentin hypersensitivity has classically consisted of using dentifrices that contain an ingredient that serves to modulate nerve depolarization and disruption of neural response to pain stimuli, as the first line of action. This method does have shortcomings in that it does not address the cause of the problem (open dentin tubules) and does not provide rapid relief.

Potassium nitrate (5%) is a well-established desensitizing agent, 5% of which has now become the widely accepted standard for application in toothpaste formulations containing fluoride. Potassium nitrate depolarizes and inactivates the pulpal nerve, thus reducing hypersensitivity and pain associated with exposed dentinal tubules. This ingredient is widely used in dentifrices claiming to reduce hypersensitivity and does have a "salty" taste but otherwise is easily formulated and is compatible with fluoride. It is the only other ingredient approved for that purpose by the FDA.

Another approach, aimed at hypersensitivity relief, uses occlusion technology to plug or seal the tubules to prevent fluid movement within the dentin tubules and the subsequent pain response. Both available technologies will be explained in detail below. Occlusion technologies include oxalates, stannous and strontium precipitates, amorphous calcium phosphate (ACP), bioactive glass, arginine bicarbonate, and others. These agents have been investigated for the treatment of hypersensitive teeth, with various degrees of clinical efficiency. For example, arginine bicarbonate–based dentifrices offer instant and lasting sensitivity relief based on a significant number of published clinical studies.

Some anti-occlusion agents, such as stannous salts or bioactive glass, along with the low-water delivery systems required to maintain their efficacy, can sometimes result in compliance issues due to taste or mouth-feel issues. Recently, a newly developed and clinically proven hypersensitivity technology that is compatible with most dentifrice formulations and is based on using a bio-adhesive agent with specially designed hydrophobic silica to occlude dentin tubules has also been introduced commercially outside the U.S.[23]

6. Non-Therapeutic Ingredients for Cosmetic Benefits

Dental calculus, or tartar, afflicts the majority of adults worldwide. Dental calculus is ossified dental plaque. It is composed primarily of calcium phosphate mineral salts deposited between what remains of previously living microorganisms, and can form above and below the gum line (supra- and subgingival). These materials typically have a rough and porous surface that provides an ideal environment for stain accumulation as well as further accumulation of plaque. Brushing and flossing can remove plaque that eventually leads to tartar; however, once formed, tartar is too hard and firmly attached to be removed with a toothbrush. Tartar buildup can be removed at the dentist office with ultrasonic tools or unique hand instruments.

A comprehensive review was given by Volpe et al.[24] describes in some detail agents that have been clinically documented to prevent tartar formation as well as the most widely accepted methodology to assess supragingival calculus based on Volpe-Manhold. This review is especially intriguing since it suggests a connection between calculus and gingival recession.

The most used tartar control agents in dentifrices as well as rinses are collectively known as condensed linear phosphates, or polyphosphates. The commercially available and best-known polyphosphates are the salts of pyrophosphates, tri-polyphosphates, and hexameta (glassy) phosphates (number of phosphorus atoms equal to 2, 3, and ~21). Polyphosphates act to inhibit the crystal growth (deposition) of the minerals (mostly calcium phosphates) in the plaque on teeth by forming a soluble complex with the calcium in the plaque, and thus control the tartar formation.

Also well known to prevent tartar are zinc salts such as zinc citrate, zinc lactate, and other soluble and insoluble zinc salts. The way the zinc ion works to prevent tartar is to poison the calcium phosphate crystal growth process by replacing calcium in the crystal lattice.

B. Mouthrinses

Mouthrinses are specially formulated solutions that are meant to be vigorously swished around the entire mouth so that the rinse comes in contact with the entire mouth—teeth, gingiva, tongue, and other oral tissues. (The authors have chosen to use the term "mouthrinse" but consider the terms "mouthwash" and "mouthrinse" as having the same definition.) There are several indications for the use of mouthrinses depending on the formulations. There are mouthrinses that are intended to help to improve oral hygiene/health (kill germs, reduce plaque, and prevent gingivitis),[25] reduce oral discomfort, strengthen enamel, provide moisture to oral tissues, and fight bad breath.[26] Oral rinses may be purchased over-the-counter (OTC) or via prescription. Mouthrinses, like dentifrices or toothpastes, can be classified as cosmetic or therapeutic, but can also be classified according to the specific end use, such as antibacterial, antigingivitis, whitening, and antiplaque. Historically, most mouthwashes have contained alcohol (6–27%) to provide the refreshing taste and help to solubilize flavor. In recent years, many major manufacturers have marketed rinses free of alcohol due the tissue irritation that occurs with alcohol and the sensitivity that some individuals have that preclude the use of alcohol.

Most of the mouthwashes have been formulated to be ready for use, while some mouthwashes (mainly in Europe) are more concentrated and are intended to be used after dilution. Mass-marketed ready-to-use mouthwashes will be the primary focus of this section.

From a usage experience point of view, a mouthwash should be a liquid of reasonable viscosity when used (not too thin or too thick), with a "pleasant" flavor. It should be safe to use on a daily basis and robust against bacterial growth during storage. Such products may be designed to foam in order to reinforce the concept of cleaning. It should be stable over the temperature range likely to be encountered during its distribution and anticipated shelf life. Although it is often a clear and single-phase solution, a few dual-phase mouthwashes, such as Dentyl pH (Fresh Breath Ltd) and Plax 2 in 1 (Colgate-Palmolive), do exist.

1. Ingredients

There is a large overlap in the ingredients used and their functions in toothpastes and mouthwashes. The approach taken in this section is to mention only those ingredients in fairly wide usage in mouthwashes.

Solvents. *Water* is the first ingredient in all ready-to-use and most concentrated mouthwashes. Purified, distilled, or deionized water is normally used to avoid interactions with other ingredients and to provide a neutral starting base for the mouthwash.

Ethyl alcohol is used in many ready-to-use mouthwashes and can be found in concentrations ranging as high as 6–27%. Alcohol helps to deliver the desired fresh-mouth feeling, and even at low levels aids in the solubilization or emulsification of the flavor, and depresses the freezing point of the formulation. It also helps to stabilize the product against microbial growth.

There was a great deal of controversy questioning whether high concentrations of alcohol were related to oral cancer. A multitude of studies have been conducted on this issue and there has been no correlation found between alcohol in mouthrinses and oral cancers.[27–29] Moreover, the American Dental Association and the U.S. Food and Drug Administration have found no indication of a causal relationship between alcohol in mouthrinses and oral cancers. Alcohol can have a drying effect on oral tissues and can be especially irritating for individuals who have xerostomia or reduced salivary flow. Individuals with alcohol-dependency problems should not use alcohol-containing mouthrinses. For persons who need to avoid alcohol-containing mouthrinses for any reason, there are nonalcoholic cosmetic mouthrinses readily available. Many of the nonalcohol mouthrinses are as effective as the alcohol-containing cosmetic mouthrinses.[30, 31]

Flavor is the reason for choice of a mouthwash by most consumers. Predominant flavor types for cosmetic type mouthwashes in the United States are mints such as spearmint, peppermint, and to a lesser extent wintergreen. These are not usually just straight oils such as peppermint *(Mentha piperita)* oil but formulated with other flavoring compounds to provide a more complex taste profile. Herbal, woody, floral, and medicinal (or phenolic) type notes are routinely added to these compounded flavors.

Flavor preferences vary widely from country to country and are even different for demographic groups of the same country. Due to the differences in flavor preferences and the relatively high cost of some flavor oils, it is necessary to carefully formulate the flavor for a product. The best way to select a flavor for a given product is by screening the prototype flavors with a target group of consumers for the product. Beyond just the taste of the flavor, the flavor may act to mask or modify the perception of bad breath, including malodor associated with "morning mouth" or the ingestion of certain types of food, such as garlic and onion. Studies are often designed to determine the effectiveness of candidate flavors in masking or altering the perception of the target odor. A common test to determine the effectiveness of a given flavor against specific malodor involves the use of judges trained in the identification of malodor.

The *essential oils/phenolics* commonly referred to in mouthwashes include thymol, eucalyptol, methyl salicylate, and menthol. Many people consider these ingredients to add a "medicinal" or "antiseptic" character to the flavor of a mouthwash.

Synthetic coolants, often the esters of menthol, have been used in products to provide a long-lasting cooling effect without the strong aftertaste associated with menthol.

Synthetic sweeteners are usually added to mouthwashes to make them have a more desirable taste. The most widely used sweeteners are sodium saccharin, sucrolase, and potassium acesulfame.

Humectants are used in mouthwashes to aid in the solubilization of flavors, to modify the mouth-feel, to add sweetness, and to increase the osmotic pressure of the mouthwash to decrease the risk of microbial growth. Humectants that have been used in recently marketed products are essentially the same as those used in toothpastes: glycerin, sorbitol, hydrogenated starch hydrolysate, propylene glycol, and xylitol. Higher levels of humectant are usually used in alcohol-free mouthwashes.

Surfactants are used in mouthwashes to emulsify or solubilize flavors and other non-water-soluble ingredients to obtain a clear product. These surfactants may also contribute to the cleansing effect of the mouthwash. Combination of the surfactants is often necessary to achieve product clarity. To ensure the cosmetic stability throughout the shelf life of the product, the formulation is evaluated for clarity and phase separation at both initial and simulated storage period under low- and high-temperature conditions.

Surfactants are widely used in mouthwash formulations. The more commonly used poloxamers are poloxamer 407, poloxamer 338, and poloxamer 124. Polysorbates, such as polysorbate 20, polysorbate 60, polysorbate 80, and steareth-20, are also used widely in mouthwash formulations. PEG-40 hydrogenated castor oil is another emulsifier used in some mouthwash products. Cationic emulsifiers were used in the past but have been abandoned in recent years due to the off-notes associated with these materials.

Anionics, for example, sodium lauryl sulfate and sodium lauryl sulfoacetate, have been used in mouthwashes, usually in combination with a nonionic. They are, however, not used in formulations containing cationic materials due to their incompatibility.

Buffers are used in some products to maintain the pH within a narrow range to help stabilize or improve the efficacy of certain ingredients. Common buffering systems include benzoic acid/sodium benzoate, phosphoric acid/sodium phosphate/disodium phosphate.

Antimicrobials. Besides killing "germs," the antimicrobials also help to reduce bad breath, plaque, and gingivitis. *Chlorhexidine digluconate* (CHX) is a cationic quaternary antimicrobial agent. It was first used in Europe in mouthrinses to treat gingivitis and periodontal disease and has now been used in a 0.12% concentration in the U.S. for many years (it is available in the U.S. by prescription). CHX is effective as an antimicrobial, as it 1) binds to oral hard and soft tissues (a process known as substantivity) and 2) causes the bacterial cell membrane to leak and allows the cytoplasm to leak out of the cell, causing cell death.

Cetylpyridium chloride (CPC) is also a cationic quaternary antimicrobial agent and binds to oral tissues, but not to the extent that CHX binds to oral tissues. CPC ruptures bacterial cell walls and destroys the cytoplasmic contents. The results of six-month studies of CPC have demonstrated a 24% reduction in gingivitis and a 16–28% reduction in dental plaque and biofilm.[32]

The *phenolic-related essential oils* used in mouthrinses include a combination of thymol, menthol, eucalyptol, and methyl salicylate. The action of the phenolic causes a disruption of the bacterial cell wall and inhibits bacterial enzymes. The substantivity of phenolic-related essential oil-containing mouthrinses is poor compared to CHX. However, these essential oil mouthrinses are antimicrobial, have antigingivitis properties and have reduced bleeding upon probing in clinical trials.

The total antimicrobial effect of a formulation is a combination of various factors: the mechanical effect of rinsing debris and microorganisms from the oral cavity, possibly enhanced by a surfactant; the effect of the antibacterial agent on the oral flora; and the possible effects of the flavor components and the alcohol, if present at a high level. Synergistic effects may also occur and should be evaluated.

Other Ingredients. *Hydrogen peroxide* (1–2%) can be used as an oxidizing/bleaching agent in mouthwashes. Because of the reactivity of hydrogen peroxide, it is not compatible with certain mouthwash ingredients, such as many flavor ingredients. Formulations with hydrogen peroxide may also require special storage conditions to minimize the degradation of the peroxide.

Chlorine dioxide, or its precursor in formulations, sodium chlorite, is used as an oxidizing agent in mouthwashes. These oxidizing materials are used primarily to fight bad breath but could also provide some antibacterial effect if properly formulated.

Zinc salts, such as zinc chloride and other soluble zinc salts, have been used in mouthwashes as a tartar control ingredient. Zinc salts are known to react with volatile sulfur compounds and therefore contribute to the breath-freshening effect. Studies have shown that they also have some antiplaque activity.

Fluoride. Sodium fluoride is compatible with most common mouthwash ingredients and can be easily formulated in mouthwashes. This effective material played an active role in inhibiting demineralization and enhancing remineralization of enamel. In the United States, fluoride-containing mouthwashes are regulated by the FDA as over-the-counter drugs only for cavity protection. Limits on the level of fluoride, formula composition, and permissible claims are outlined in the FDA anti-caries monograph and should be reviewed and followed carefully during formulation development.

Preservatives are used in mouthwashes, especially alcohol free mouthwashes, to help maintain the micro-robustness during manufacturing process and throughout the product shelf life. Common preservatives used in mouthwashes include parabens (methyl and propyl-paraben), potassium sorbate, and sodium benzoate. Most of the preservatives have an optimal pH range for the best preservation effect. It is important to take this into consideration when developing mouthwash formulation.

There are many ingredients that are occasionally used in mouthwashes. These include a number of salts, polymers, surfactants, antibacterial agents, and natural extracts. One of these ingredients is tetrasodium pyrophosphate. Tetrasodium pyrophosphate is normally used in mouthwash for its anti-tartar and stain-prevention effect. Another ingredient is xanthan gum, which is used for its film-forming properties to stabilize the foam generated by the surfactant. Sodium bicarbonate or baking soda is used in a few mouthwashes for its malodor-reducing properties.

FORMULATION EXAMPLES OF MOUTHWASHES

Alcohol-Free Mouthwash

Ingredient	**%**
Water	86.01
Benzoic acid	0.04
Sodium benzoate	0.15
Poloxamer 407	1.25
Glycerin	12.00
Sodium saccharin	0.05
FD&C Blue No. 1	0.0002
Flavor	0.25
Polysorbate 20	0.25

Alcohol-Containing Mouthwash

Ingredient	**%**
Water	76.18
Glycerin	8.00
Sodium benzoate	0.10
Benzoic acid	0.04
Sodium saccharin	0.08
Cetylpyridinium chloride	0.05
FD&C Blue No. 1	0.0002
SDA alcohol 38-B	15.00
Flavor	0.25
Polysorbate 80	0.30

2. Manufacture

Mouthwashes are generally prepared in three steps. In step one, water-soluble/miscible ingredients including actives, surfactants, some humectant, and colors are dissolved in water. In step two, flavor is dissolved in the remainder of humectant, such as propylene glycol, as a premix. Step three, premix is added to the aqueous phase and emulsified to form a homogenous solution. The final step in production is filtration through a series of filters to ensure that no particulates are present in the final products.

3. Packaging

Both ready-to-use and concentrate mouthwashes are packed in bottles. Historically most mouthwashes were packed in glass with a re-sealable cap. Glass was considered to be nonreactive and provided "perfect" barrier properties. The trend in the beverage industry toward lighter-weight and more break-resistant plastic containers has influenced the manufacturers of mouthwash to adopt plastic bottles. Today the majority of mouthwashes are sold in plastic bottles with a re-sealable plastic cap. The resins of choice for the bottle are polyethylene terephthalate (PET) and polyvinyl chloride (PVC). Some high-density polyethylene, exotic resins and coextruded bottles also exist. In general, PET offers better product transparency than PVC.

In the United States, FDA regulation requires "tamper-evident" packaging for mouthwashes, and Consumer Product Safety Commission regulation requires child-resistant caps for certain fluoride-containing mouthwashes.

6.18.2 ORAL HYGIENE AIDS

A. Manual toothbrush

The most often-asked questions of dental hygienists and dentists are "What toothpaste should I use?" and "What toothbrush should I use?" The professional answer to both questions will depend on which of these products best fits the patient's needs. For toothbrushes, there is an added dimension—which one will be the most effective for the patient, with regard to the thorough removal of dental plaque biofilm. The most fundamental point regarding dental health and dental plaque biofilm is that it must be mechanically removed. Dentifrices and mouthrinses are adjunctive and can certainly be bactericidal. None, however are 100% effective at killing the oral bacteria and removing the strongly adherent acquired pellicle (the pellicle is the first organic film to form on the tooth surface prior to the formation of dental plaque.

1. Historical Perspective

Since ancient times people have made devices for cleaning their teeth. Chew sticks, known as miswaks or *siwaks* sticks, were made of twigs from the arak tree and were some of the first known toothbrushes, made by the Babylonians as early as 3500 BCE. The invention of the bristle toothbrush was credited to a Chinese emperor in the seventh century. Stiff boar's hair was used as bristles and attached to bamboo or bone handles. The toothbrushes were imported to Europe by travelers to China. The Europeans found the boar bristles to be too stiff and caused their gums to bleed. The Chinese altered their toothbrush by substituting horse hair for boar's hair. Toothbrushes were not mass-produced in Europe until 1780 when they were introduced by William Addie of Clerkenwald, England.

The first U.S. patent for a toothbrush was granted in 1857 to H.N. Wadsworth, but toothbrushes were not mass-produced in the U.S. until after the Civil War, around 1885. Inventors have been actively developing new designs ever since. Wallace H. Carothere worked for DuPont Laboratories and invented nylon in 1937. By 1938 nylon-bristle toothbrushes were being marketed in the U.S. The first nylon-bristle toothbrush was marketed as Dr. West's Miracle Toothbrush. The Prophylactic Brush, made by the Florence Manufacturing Company of Massachusetts, was the first rival to the Dr. West's toothbrush. After World War II, toothbrushes were available all across the U.S.

2. Importance of Toothbrush Features

The modern manual toothbrush has gone through a tremendous evolution. Consumers can choose from a large array of toothbrush handle shapes, sizes and colors, bristle profiles, and bristle stiffness. To satisfy their individual preferences, consumers can choose from many different product features.

The effectiveness of a manual toothbrush is, to a different degree, dependent on (1) the design and materials the toothbrush is made of, and (2) how well the patient uses the toothbrush. If the patient has had toothbrushing instructions from a dental hygienist or dentist and has had their toothbrushing effectiveness evaluated during maintenance visits, the patient is more likely to be successful at thorough dental plaque biofilm removal.

The patient, and how he or she uses the toothbrush, is critical to successful brushing. That stated, there are some features of toothbrush design that have been universally accepted by dental healthcare providers. Importantly, a soft to ultra-soft bristled toothbrush is the most important feature for thorough dental plaque biofilm removal. Softer bristles will get into spaces, pits, and fissures where hard- or even medium-bristled brushes will pass over the high portions of the tooth. Additionally, soft to ultra-soft bristle toothbrushes are much less likely to cause tissue trauma or discomfort. This is especially important to the patient that has gingivitis or periodontitis or sensitive teeth or gingiva. If the bristles are stiff and cause trauma to tissue that is already sensitive, the patient will be less likely to thoroughly remove the dental plaque biofilm.

The American Dental Association has safety and acceptance guidelines for manufacturers to obtain the Seal of Acceptance. The American Dental Association has incorporated the International Standard Organization's standards for manual and powered toothbrushes with their own standards to formulate the guidelines for the Seal of Acceptance. Some of these standards include:

- toothbrush bristles must be soft
- the bristles must be free of sharp or jagged edges
- there are specific guidelines regarding the number of bristles in each tuft and requirements for bristle retention
- manufacturers have many creative handle designs; however, the only requirement from the ADA is that the handle be durable under normal use.

With the emphasis on having patients use soft-bristled toothbrushes, these are the factors that determine toothbrush stiffness:

- the number of filaments in each tuft
- the number of tufts
- the type of material used to make the bristles
- the length of the bristles
- the diameter of the bristles.

B. Powered Toothbrush

1. Historical Perspective

Like manual toothbrushes, powered toothbrushes have also undergone enormous changes since they were first introduced. There were several "powered toothbrushes" patented as early as 1885 that were not actually "powered" by electricity.

The first actual electrically powered toothbrush was made available to consumers in the U.S. after World War II. E.R. Squibb & Sons manufactured the *Broxodent* in 1960. In 1961, General Electric produced the first rechargeable cordless toothbrush. These early electric toothbrushes had simple actions. The Broxodent had a reciprocating back-and-forth motion and the General Electric toothbrush had an accurate motion. Dental hygienists and dentists did not immediately embrace these electric toothbrushes. Most often, dental hygienists and dentists recommended these toothbrushes to patients who had a physical impairment or had orthodontic appliances or some other type of need.[33] There were fears that patients would brush too vigorously. Early clinical research revealed no difference in brushing with a manual versus and electric toothbrush. Importantly, later studies indicated that the control of gingivitis was improved with a powered toothbrush.

With the latest generations of powered toothbrushes that range from sonic to ultrasonic, there is ample evidence that when used correctly, powered toothbrushes will remove dental plaque biofilm and reduce gingivitis equivalent to or better than manual toothbrushes. It must be emphasized that no matter what type of toothbrush is being utilized, it is the user that makes the most important impact on the efficacy and thoroughness of cleaning. Following the instructions of the manufacturer and of dental professionals is of utmost importance.

2. Types of Powered Toothbrushes

a. Range of Products

An electric toothbrush is a toothbrush where the motion of the brush head is driven rapidly by electric power. In its earliest generation, the device was plugged into regular outlets and powered by AC current. The advent of the battery-operated design removed both the physical constraint and safety concerns of the AC-powered devices in the bathroom environment.

The basic **battery-powered toothbrushes** are similar in design to regular manual toothbrushes, where the brush head delivers similar reciprocal brushing actions. The power is provided by common AA or AAA batteries.

The rechargeable type is where the device is equipped with a cradle that plugs into the wall for the battery recharge. The cradle functions as the charging base using metal tabs to connect to the rechargeable batteries. In the more advanced designs, power is being transferred through contactless induction. The brush component is usually detachable from the main body and is replaceable when the bristles are worn. Rechargeable electric toothbrushes are, in general, more advanced in the degree of cleaning actions. They use dynamic motions such as oscillating-rotating or sonic technology to provide more effective cleaning and plaque removal.

With the innovation of electronic technology, the powered toothbrush advanced beyond the basic simulation of manual motion. The latest models include the Colgate® ProClinical® Powered Toothbrushes with distinct multidirectional cleaning action. One model, the A1500, combines high-frequency mechanism, electronic sensors, and an ergonomic handle design that intelligently and automatically adjusts the speed and the motion of the brush head corresponding to its position in the mouth. Without the need of specific training, consumers gained a stronger brushing experience and better cleaning of the teeth and gums with this unique sensing and control technology.

b. Action

Most power toothbrushes are simple to use, but quite different than manual toothbrushes. Unlike manual toothbrushes, which require the patient to generate the action of the toothbrush, power toothbrushes generate the bristle action and the patient needs to merely move the toothbrush around the mouth—tooth to tooth, ensuring that each tooth is cleaned thoroughly. Power toothbrushes have a variety of ways that the bristles move in the head of the toothbrush. Examples include:

- Head is stationary; each tuft of bristles moves in counter-rotational directions
- Rotating-oscillating head; stationary bristles

- Rotating-oscillating-pulsating
- Oscillating-pulsating-pivoting
- Rotary head with interchangeable heads that include a brush with a single tuft of bristles, a hollow-cup brush, and an elongated brush tip that rotates
- Side-to-side action
- Multidirectional cleaning action

c. Sonic and Ultrasonic

Power toothbrushes can be further classified according to the speed of vibration. Sonic toothbrushes vibrate in the audible range of 30,000 brush (260 Hz) strokes per minute. Ultrasonic power toothbrushes have a high-frequency bristle motion (18,000,000 strokes per minute) at ultrasonic vibration that produces greater than 20,000 Hz.

d. Additional Features

Newer products also feature a wide variety of computer-assisted capabilities. These features include timers, a variety of settings that range from a slower speed for brushing up to higher speeds meant for stain removal and whitening, and digital screens that inform the patient that they are brushing too hard or brushing incorrectly in some fashion or not brushing long enough.

C. Interdental Cleaning Devices

The one shortcoming of the toothbrush, whether it is powered to manual, is that none of them are made so that the user can adequately clean between the teeth. The lack of any physiological interdental cleaning underscores the need and importance of interdental cleaning devices.

1. Importance of Interdental Cleaning

Despite the mantra of "brush and floss" from dental professionals, studies tracking in-home use of dental floss indicate that only 2–10% of patients regularly performed acceptable flossing and most did not floss on a daily basis.[34]

The interdental papilla, the gingival tissue that lies between the teeth, has a physiological shortcoming that makes it more vulnerable to the effects of dental plaque biofilm and bacterial endotoxins. That shortcoming is a col area that is non-keratinized (the col area is the area of the gingiva that is anatomically in the center from the facial side [cheek side] of the gingiva to the lingual [tongue-side] of the gingiva). It does not have the tougher, keratinized tissue that covers the outside surfaces of the gingiva. This col tissue is very susceptible to being ulcerated due to endotoxins and inflammatory reactions due to the bacterial challenge. If dental plaque biofilm is not removed at least once every 24 hours, that nonkeratinized gingiva is exposed to material that will cause it to break down and succumb to inflammation and chronic periodontal disease. Further, this interdental plaque is the source of some of the volatile sulfur-containing compounds from bacteria that cause halitosis. If patients do not believe this, all they have to do is floss their teeth and then smell the floss! They will be instant believers!

2. Dental Floss—The Shortcomings

The highest form of scientific evidence is the systematic review. There have been some excellent systematic reviews on the use of dental floss.[34–37] The information revealed in these studies is very important, but may not come as a surprise to dental professionals:

- The strength and quality of evidence in most randomized clinical trials on dental flossing is very low.[36]
- There is insufficient evidence that dental floss reduces plaque.[40]
- There are no studies that indicate that the use of dental floss reduces the risk of dental caries.[35]
- The quality of evidence to support the theory that flossing and toothbrushing reduce gingivitis is very low.[36]
- When dental professionals flossed patients' teeth, significant benefits were seen that were not seen when patients flossed their own teeth.[37]
- Many individuals do not know how to floss properly or have the dexterity to do so; for subjects researched that did use floss with toothbrushing, there was no added benefit to the flossing.[35, 36]

It makes sense that if the interdental spaces are too wide for floss to contact both sides of the interproximal surfaces of the teeth, then the floss is not going to be effective at removing the dental plaque biofilm. It is logical that any interdental cleaner that is wide enough to fill the interproximal space and reach to the interproximal surfaces will be effective in interproximal plaque removal. Dental hygienists and dentists need to be responsible for assisting patients to find the best interdental cleaning method to meet their need.[38]

3. Interdental Brushes

Interdental brushes are one of the most efficacious interdental cleaning aids available. They are available in various sizes; the very smallest interdental brushes (in diameter) will normally fit a normal, healthy interdental space that is tight. There are larger sizes and importantly, they are available in conical and cylindrical shapes. Interdental brushes are available with nylon bristles and also with elastomeric "fingers" that work similarly to bristles.

4. Additional Interdental Cleaning Aids

There are a multitude of interdental cleaning aids available, and dental hygienists and dentists must be careful in guiding patients to the aids that will be most useful for them—the recommendations should be patient-centered. It is important that dental healthcare professionals be aware of the scientific evidence behind the interdental aids and ensure that the patient has been instructed on the correct use of the interdental aid. The interdental aid that will be most successful is the one that will adequately fill the interproximal space (embrasure) without causing tissue trauma. Fortunately there are numerous types, shapes, and sizes of interdental aids available:

- End-tufted brushes
- Floss threaders
- Interdental cleaners with elastomeric “fingers”
- Interproximal (interdental brushes)
- Powered flossers
- Rubber-tip stimulators
- Soft wooden sticks
- Textured flosses
- Toothpicks
- Waterflossers (oral irrigators)

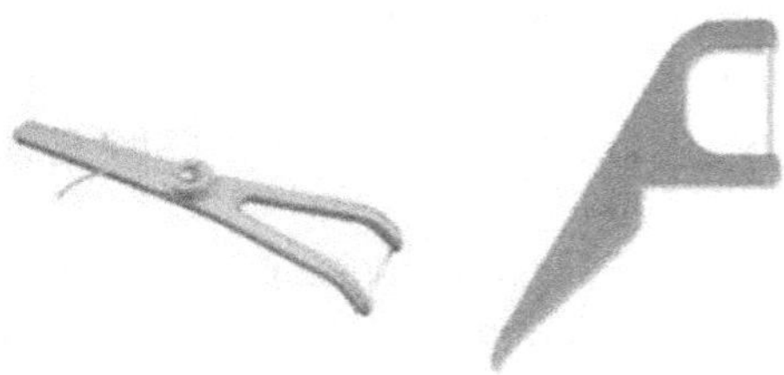

Figure 2: Floss holders

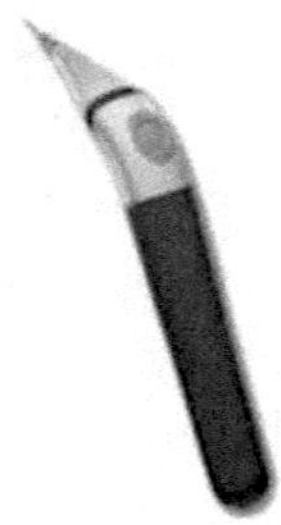

Figure 3: Powered Flosser

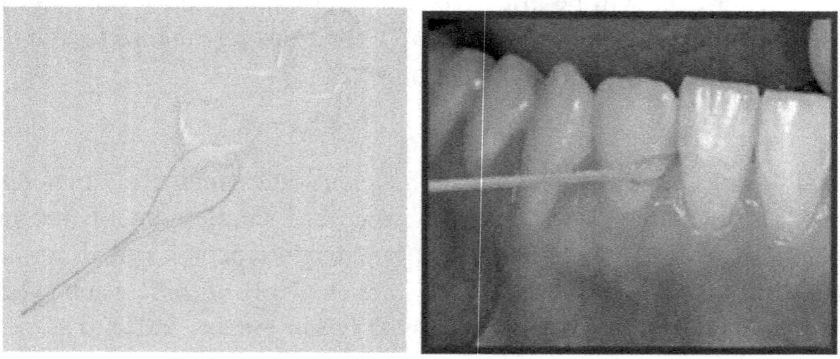

Figure 4: Floss Threader

Figures 2–4: illustrate various interdental cleaning aids.

SUMMARY

Oral health is taken much more seriously now that it is recognized that an unhealthy mouth with millions of disease-causing bacteria is related to systemic diseases. It is quite logical that the presence of chronic inflammation lasting for years with soft tissue and bone destruction and tissue death is going to have effects on other parts of the body and body systems. Other healthcare professionals are realizing that the mouth is connected to the rest of the body. Clearly there will be research that continues to explore the relationship between oral health and overall systemic health.

There has never been a time where so much has been known about what causes dental diseases, and this knowledge is accompanied by a wealth of products that can support successful oral preventive self-care. The use of fluoride and oral health education has worked and the payoff is tangible: senior citizens, even in nursing homes, have their teeth. The future of dental health has never been better as long as citizens of all ages have access to care.

REFERENCES

1. U.S. Department of Health and Human Services. Oral health in America: a report of the Surgeon General. Rockville, MD: Department of Health and Human Services, National Institute of Dental and Craniofacial Research, National Institutes of Health, 2000. Available from: http://www.surgeongeneral.gov/library/oralhealth/
2. Centers for Disease Control and Prevention Report. Oral health: preventing cavities, gum disease, and oral cancers. 2004
3. Barnes, CM. Managing Incipient and Hidden Caries, *Dental Clinics of North America*, 2005 (4)795–814.
4. Centers for Disease Control and Prevention, Division of Oral Health, Best Practices Report of the Association of State and Territorial Dental Directors, 2003. http://www.cdc.gov/OralHealth, accessed June 11, 2014
5. Centers for Disease Control and Prevention, Division of Oral Health. Oral Health Program: Strategic Planning for 2011–2014. http://www.cdc.gov/OralHealth/strageticplan.Accessed June 11, 2014
6. www.mindfloss.com, accessed June 8, 2014. National Retail Federation/American Pet **Product** Association
7. American Academy of Cosmetic Dentistry. AACD State of the Cosmetic Dentistry Industry 2011, http://www.aacd.com/, assessed June 8, 2014.
8. AACD 2007 survey http://www.aacd.com/, assessed June 8, 2014.

9. Kissmegoodnight. http://www.kissmegoodnight.com/bad-breath/bad-breath-statistics.shtm, accessed June 6, 2014.
10. Clark GT, Nachnani S, Messagi DV: Detecting and treating oral and non-oral malodors. *J Calif Dent Assoc* 25(2) : 133–145, 1997.
11. Scully G et all: Breath odor: etiopathogenesis, assessment and management., *Euro J Oral Sci* 105: 287–293, 1997.
12. Semann R et al: Effectiveness of mechanical tongue cleaning on oral levels of volatile sulfuric compounds, *J Am Dent Assn* 132: 1263–1267, 2001.
13. Silood CJL, Grootveld, MC, Lynch E: A multifactorial investigation of the ability of oral health care products to alleviate oral malodour. *J Clin Periodontol* 28: 634–641, 2001.
14. Nurata T, Yamaga T, Lida T, Miyazaki H, Yaegaki K. Classification and examination of halitosis. *International Dent J* 52 Suppl 3: 181–186, 2002.
15. Barnes CM. Interdental cleaning success. *Dimensions in Dental Hygiene*; 11(9): 19–22, September 2013.
16. Federal Interagency Forum on Aging-Related Statistics. 2012. http://www.agingstats.gov/Main_Site/Data/Data_2012.aspx, accessed July 27, 2014.
17. The aging mouth and how to keep it younger. The Harvard Medical School Family Health Guide. http://www.health.harvard.edu/fhg/updates/the-aging-mouth.shtml, accessed June 11, 2014.
18. Dental Hygiene Statistics, Statistic Brain, www.statisticbrain.com/dental-hygiene-statistics, accessed July 27, 2014.
19. Cosmetics and your health fact sheet. www.womenshealth.gov/publications/../cosmetics-your-health.html accessed July 27, 2014.
20. Prencipe M, Masters G, Thomas KP, Norfleet M, Squeezing Out a Better Toothpaste, *CHEMTECH*, December 1995
21. Anticaries Drug products for Over-the-Counter Human Use,, Federal Register, 60, 52474–52510, Oct 6., 1005
22. Panagakos FS, Volpe AR, Petrone ME, Morrison, Jr. BM, DeVizio W, Davies RM, Proskin HM, Advanced Oral Antibacterial/Anti-inflammatory Technology: A Comprehensive Review of the Clinical Benefits of a Triclosan/Copolymer/Fluoride Dentifrice, *J Clin Dent.* 2014;25(Suppl):S1–30.

23. Zaidel L, Patel R, Mello S, Heu R, Stranick M, Chopra S, Prencipe M, Anti-hypersensitivity Mechanism of Action for a Dentifrice Containing 0.3% Triclosan, 2% PVM/MA copolymer, 0.243% NaF, and Specially-designed Silica , *American Journal of Dentistry*, Vo. 24, pp 1A–32A, July 2011

24 Volpre RA, Petrone, ME, Davies RM, A Review of Calculus Clinical Efficacy Studies, *The International Journal of Applied Dental Research*, Vol IV, No.3, pp 71–81, 1993.

25. Silverman S, Wilder R: Antimicrobial mouthrinse as part of a comprehensive oral care regimen. Safety and compliance factors. *JADA* 2006, 137 (11), 22S–26S.

26. Fedorowicz Z, Aljufairi H, Nasser M, Outhouse TL, Pedrazzi V: Mouthrinses for the treatment of halitosis. *Cochrane Database Syst Rev.* 2008 Oct 8;(4):CD006701.

27. Lemos CA Jr, Villoria GE: Reviewed evidence about the safety of the daily use of alcohol-based mouthrinses. Braz Oral Res, 2008, 22 Suppl 1: 24–31.

28. Werner CW, Seymour RA: Are alcohol containing mouthwashes safe? Brit Dent J 2009, 207 (10): E19, 488–489.

29. Mascarenhas AK: Inconclusive evidence to suggest that alcohol-containing mouthwash increases the risk of oropharyngeal cancer. *J Evid Base Dent Prac*, 2005, 4: 249–250.

30. Recovering Alcoholics and Mouthwash. Alcohol Rehab.com http://alcoholrehab.com/alcoholism/recovering-alcoholics-and-mouthwash.html , accessed June 29, 2014.

31. Anyanwu OC, Baugh KK, Bennett SB, Johnson JM, Madlock RL, Pollard NE, Chikwem JO: comparison of the effectiveness of alcohol-containing vs. non-alcohol containing mouthwash. Linc Univ J of Sci, 2011, 2(1): 7–12.

32. Lobene RR, Kashket S, Soparkar PM, Shloss J, Sabine ZM. The effect of cetylpridinium chloride on human plaque bacteria and gingivitis. *Pharmacol Ther Dent.* 1979; 4(1):33–47.

33. Bowen D. An evidenced –based review of powered toothbrushes. *Compend Oral Hyg* 9(1): 3–18. 2002.

34. Hujoel PP, Cunha-CruzJ, Banting DW, Loesche WJ. Dental flossing and interproximal caries: a systematic review. J Dent Res 2006, 85: 298–305.

35. Sambunjak D, Nickerson JW, Poklepovic T. flossing for the management of periodontal diseases and dental caries in adults. Cochrane Database System Rev. 2011,:7: CD008829.

36. Bader HI. Floss or die: implications for dental professionals. *Dent Today* 1998 17: 76–82

37. Berchier CE, Slot DE, Hap S, Van der Weijden GA. The efficacy of dental floss in addition to a toothbrush on plaque and parameters of gingival inflammation: a systematic review. Int J Dent Hyg 2008, 6: 265–279

38. Barnes CM. Interdental cleaning success. Dimensions Dent Hyg 2013; 11(9): 19–22.

www.ingramcontent.com/pod-product-compliance
Lightning Source LLC
LaVergne TN
LVHW011128300926
849160LV00008B/561
* 9 7 8 0 8 2 0 6 0 1 9 9 1 *